NEW DIRECTIONS FOR STUDENT SERVICES

Margaret J. Barr, *Northwestern University*
EDITOR-IN-CHIEF

M. Lee Upcraft, *The Pennsylvania State University*
ASSOCIATE EDITOR

Successful Drug and Alcohol Prevention Programs

Eileen V. Coughlin
Western Washington University

EDITOR

Number 67, Fall 1994

JOSSEY-BASS PUBLISHERS
San Francisco

SUCCESSFUL DRUG AND ALCOHOL PREVENTION PROGRAMS
Eileen V. Coughlin (ed.)
New Directions for Student Services, no. 67
Margaret J. Barr, Editor-in-Chief
M. Lee Upcraft, Associate Editor

Microfilm copies of issues and articles are available in 16mm and 35mm, as well as microfiche in 105mm, through University Microfilms Inc., 300 North Zeeb Road, Ann Arbor, Michigan 48106-1346.

LC 85-644751   ISSN 0164-7970   ISBN 0-7879-9996-2

NEW DIRECTIONS FOR STUDENT SERVICES is part of The Jossey-Bass Higher and Adult Education Series and is published quarterly by Jossey-Bass Inc., Publishers, 350 Sansome Street, San Francisco, California 94104-1342. Second-class postage paid at San Francisco, California, and at additional mailing offices. POSTMASTER: Send address changes to New Directions for Teaching and Learning, Jossey-Bass Inc., Publishers, 350 Sansome Street, San Francisco, California 94104-1342.

SUBSCRIPTIONS for 1994 cost $47.00 for individuals and $62.00 for institutions, agencies, and libraries.

EDITORIAL CORRESPONDENCE should be sent to the Editor-in-Chief, Margaret J. Barr, 633 Clark Street, 2-219, Evanston, Illinois 60208-1103.

Cover photograph by Wernher Krutein/PHOTOVAULT © 1990.

Manufactured in the United States of America. Nearly all Jossey-Bass books, jackets, and periodicals are printed on recycled paper that contains at least 50 percent recycled waste, including 10 percent postconsumer waste. Many of our materials are also printed with vegetable-based inks; during the printing process, these inks emit fewer volatile organic compounds (VOCs) than petroleum-based inks. VOCs contribute to the formation of smog.

CONTENTS

EDITOR'S NOTES

In the past twenty-five years, prevention policies and procedures related to alcohol abuse and illicit drug use in higher education have vacillated with societal norms. These norms have influenced the context in which student services are delivered. A part of this context has been the maturing of the relationship between students and the higher education institutions that serve them.

During this same time, the correlation between alcohol and drug abuse and campus crime, exposure to sexually transmitted diseases, relationship problems, accidents, and increased potential for academic failure have been inextricably linked. In response to these concerns, new federal regulations were enacted to ensure the development of programs to prevent alcohol abuse and other drug use (Public law 101–226 section 1213). On most campuses, student services professionals have provided the primary leadership for implementation of these prevention programs.

The purpose of this volume is to explore the extent of the current problem and to present the latest alcohol and other drug prevention techniques in higher education. The authors recognize that the delivery and format of prevention programs must be tailored to the campus environment in which they exist. Therefore, the work included was selected to stimulate new ways of thinking about campus prevention activities with the understanding that creative application of these techniques is essential to meeting the needs of the campus culture in which those services are delivered.

Chapter One introduces the problem from both a quantitative and an anecdotal perspective. Included in this chapter are liability concerns and a delineation of the students who are at greatest risk. This is followed by Chapter Two, in which Cheryl Presley, Philip Meilman, and Julie Padgett present myths and facts that are critical to the education of faculty and administrators.

No one would deny that acquiring the support of the president or chancellor is a valued asset in prevention programs. In Chapter Three, Paul Gianini, president of Valencia Community College in Florida, and Ruth Nicholson identify avenues for relating prevention activities to the issues of most concern to presidents.

A variety of prevention approaches are presented in Chapters Four, Five, and Six. These chapters describe programs that have immediate practical application for prevention practitioners. In Chapter Four, Diane Edwards and Patricia Leonard stretch our thinking by approaching prevention through the symbols, artifacts, and rituals adopted by student subcultures. In Chapter Five, Emily Wadsworth, John Hoeppel, and Kipp Hassell give an account of an alternative model in which faculty teach prevention activities across the curriculum. Chapter Six describes the characteristics of successful programs with examples included from a variety of campuses researched and reported by Beverly Mills-Novoa.

The final two chapters offer a strategic planning and assessment tool along with additional resources for practitioners. Beverly Mills-Novoa and I encourage the use of quantitative and qualitative assessment to ensure a continuous process of program improvement. Chapter Seven includes a qualitative assessment tool to achieve this goal. In the last chapter, I provide some closing thoughts along with a brief annotated bibliography.

This volume was written primarily by administrators and faculty practitioners whose time and energy have been devoted to directly serving students through a long-term commitment to developing healthy campus cultures. I would like to thank these authors for their continued work in this difficult area of student affairs. I would also like to recognize the contribution of Ronald Bucknam, director of the Fund for the Improvement of Postsecondary Education, whose creative administration has supported many of the programs presented in this volume. I am also grateful to Marti Weinzinger, who organized and managed the manuscript details, and to Thomas Canepa for the graphics included in the volume.

Eileen V. Coughlin
Editor

EILEEN V. COUGHLIN is vice president for student affairs and dean of academic support services at Western Washington University, Bellingham. She was also director of the qualitative evaluation project presented in chapters Six and Seven.

The increased need for leadership in alcohol and other drug abuse prevention in higher education is evident in both the quantitative and anecdotal evidence from students. The number of students at risk and the financial and legal implications of inaction make prevention an imperative for student affairs.

Students at Risk: Alcohol and Drug Prevention in Context

Eileen V. Coughlin

The problem of alcohol and other drug abuse on American college campuses has become increasingly complex. Not only has the heterogeneity of the student population increased significantly, but legal, social, and developmental issues have also intensified. This is evident in the interaction of alcohol and other drugs with difficult social problems such as AIDS, sexual assault, and criminal and civil liabilities. In addition, there is conflict between the legal drinking age and the responsible drinking philosophy used on many campuses. This conflict has challenged administrators to do battle with themselves in trying to balance violations of the law against their respect for students as adults.

To add insult to injury, one of the most recent drugs on the underground market, "cat" or methcathinone, was reproduced in a laboratory in a residence hall at Northern Michigan University in the early 1990s. Although it never became popular among students at the university, it did create a mini-epidemic in the rural upper peninsula of Michigan and appeared as far away as Seattle (Anderson and Binstein, 1993). The encroachment of this type of drug manufacturing onto the college campus is an assault on the values of higher education.

For student affairs administrators, there is no escape. "The effects of problems with alcohol and other drugs are sometimes subtle, sometimes extravagant, and always debilitating, both to the individual and to the community of which he or she is part" (Donovan, 1990, p. 24). The increased mental capacities of those in the higher education community may foster the development of highly sophisticated individualized denial systems that create greater barriers to recognizing students at risk. Donovan (1990) warned that "Such problems have special poignancy in an intellectual community where, despite all evidence to the contrary, hope still exists that troubled individuals will somehow see the difficulties they are facing and get a grip on themselves" (Donovan, 1990, p. 24). The focus of attention on alcohol and other substance abuse problems on college campuses has been on the individual abuser, with a hope that by some miracle the rest of us might elude responsibility.

This chapter is intended to provide a synopsis of recent research on the pattern of college student alcohol and other drug use along with anecdotal evidence related to its impact. In addition, a brief historical perspective is presented in order to better understand the more recent legislative changes that have affected the prevention of alcohol and other drug abuse. Following this background is a review of students at particular risk of the negative consequences of alcohol and other drug abuse.

Research on Student Use

Before reviewing recent research on college student use of alcohol and other drugs, it is important to consider some of the statistical comparisons and context for the changes that have occurred. Perhaps the most important caution was provided by Johnston, O'Malley, and Bachman in 1989 as a part of their longitudinal study, *Drug Use, Drinking, and Smoking: National Survey Results from High School, College, and Young Adults Populations 1975–1988*. "Despite the improvements in recent years, it is still true that this nation's high school students and other young adults show a level of involvement with illicit drugs which is greater than can be found in any other industrialized nation in the world. Even by longer-term historical standards in this country, these rates remain extremely high" (Johnston, O'Malley, and Bachman, 1989, p. 15).

Some recent statistical comparisons provide a sobering perspective. Forty-one percent of college students get drunk versus 34 percent of their noncollege counterparts. Students spend more on alcohol than the collective cost of operating campus libraries, scholarships, and fellowships in the United States—$4.2 billion annually. It is projected that an equal number of college students will die of alcohol-related causes as will obtain masters and doctoral degrees (Wertz, 1991). After reviewing the literature, Gonzales and Broughton (1986, p. 49) concluded, "a disproportionate share of alcohol-related problems can be found on the college campus." In other words, the campus culture may facilitate the abuse of alcohol by individual students.

There are two longitudinal studies that provide some cause for hope. The first of these is the work of Johnston, O'Malley, and Bachman that covers drug and alcohol use from 1975 to 1992. The proportion of college students using illicit drugs declined significantly between 1980 and 1991, from 56 percent to 29 percent. This trend paralleled the decline in both high school and noncollege peers during the same period. However, college students showed less decline in heavy drinking than the other two populations during the same time: there was a 13.5 percent decline in heavy drinking among high school seniors, a 10.7 percent decline in nonstudents, and only a 2.2 percent decline in heavy drinking among college students between 1981 and 1992 (Johnston, O'Malley, and Bachman, 1993). The Core survey is the second longitudinal study of relevance and it is presented in greater detail in the chapter *Facts and Myths*. This research supports the positive impact of drug prevention programs. Institutions that participated in both the pre- and postsurvey demonstrated a slight decrease in the amount of alcohol use per student, from 4.95 to 4.80 drinks per week. In addition, the research indicated that students exposed to FIPSE-funded prevention programs reported fewer episodes of binge drinking.

In addition, the 1984–1985 National Study of Substance Use and Abuse Habits of College Student-Athletes reflects similar trends among athletes. A 1992–1993 replication of the original study found that athletes, particularly football players, had significantly reduced their use of anabolic steroids. Furthermore, the use of amphetamines, barbiturates, and pain medications all decreased. However, during this same time, binge drinking reported among athletes increased from 35 percent in 1985 to 47 percent in 1993 (NCAA, 1993).

The data related to alcohol abuse corroborate the views of student affairs administrators who indicated that they either saw no change in the existing alcohol problems on their campuses or saw an increase in problems. Despite prevention efforts of the early 1980s, a 1988 study reported in the *Chronicle of Higher Education* revealed that "35 percent of student-affairs administrators thought campus problems involving alcohol had increased in the past several years, and 41 percent saw no change" (Magner, 1988a, p. A35). In other words, under the leadership of mostly student affairs professionals, higher education has simultaneously made progress in helping to reduce illicit drug use among students and at the same time seen little change in alcohol abuse.

Unfortunately, any sense of optimism in the decline of illicit drug use has been overshadowed by the most recent *Monitoring the Future* data. This research by Johnston, Bachman, and O'Malley was publicly reported in a news release on January 31, 1994. According to this report, "Drug use among American young people has been making a clear comeback in the past two years" (University of Michigan, 1994, p. 1). This report includes research on high school seniors, tenth graders, and eighth graders. The data indicate 3 to 4 percent one-year increases in marijuana use, followed by smaller increases in hallucinogens, LSD, and inhalants. Based on the 1992–1994 data, Johnston stated, "Certainly the combination of drugs now growing in popularity—marijuana, LSD, and amphetamines—is reminiscent of what was popular in the early days of the drug epidemic. Other drugs then followed in popularity" (University of Michigan, 1994, p. 3).

The students represented in this sample include future college students. In fact, the 24th Annual Survey of High Achievers (juniors and seniors in high school with a B average and above) confirmed similar drug and alcohol use by high achievers. Paul Krouse, publisher of the reference book, was quoted as saying "AIDS doesn't scare them. Pregnancy does, but not enough to make them take precautions consistently. And drinking is a way of life, even behind the wheel" (Feldman, 1993, p. 1).

Anecdotal Evidence

The anecdotal data are even more chilling. An excerpt in the March 3, 1993, edition of the *Chronicle of Higher Education* quotes a college senior who spoke about his experience as a fraternity member. "I left not because of any moral awakening, but because I could barely stay sober long enough to write my name. This was my problem, not the system's" ("Quotable," 1993, p. B5). The documented benefits of fraternity membership, including a higher graduation rate (Astin, 1975, 1992), suggest that they deserve our continued administrative support. However, a recent study of two fraternities' cultures indicates that "alcohol is a key element in a complicated system of reward and sanctions used by fraternities to socialize new comers" (Kuh and Arnold, 1993, p. 34).

In the words of one college sophomore who has experienced tragedy among her peers, "It is often easy to pinpoint the college drinking problem on a certain group such as athletes or fraternities. Drinking is in every dorm on every campus whether we see it or not. It has become sociable and a way of being accepted. It is a major problem and I wonder how many accidents, DUIs and even deaths it will take for people to realize it is a problem that grows bigger every day" (Mayes, personal interview, 1994).

Who Is Responsible?

Who is responsible for the effects of alcohol and other substance abuse on college and university campuses across the country? This question conjures images of Bil Keane's *Family Circus* cartoons. Keane captures the essence of individual and institutional denial with his infamous NOT ME ghost. In these cartoons, the NOT ME ghost appears whenever Billy, Dolly, Jeffy, or P. J. get into trouble and the loaded question is asked: Who is responsible for this?

The NOT ME ghost roams not only among students, but also among administrators, parents, faculty, and society. Perhaps this is a reflection of our feelings of helplessness or our recognition that it could just as easily have been us. However, too much time is spent trying to find someone to blame rather than recognizing that each member of the higher education community plays a part in designing and maintaining a healthy environment. In other words, it is both an individual problem and a cultural problem. The exorcism of the NOT ME ghost on college campuses is the first step toward individual and systemic change.

In an effort to better understand the NOT ME ghost of alcohol use, we must first stop to listen. We may be aware of the daily messages our campus community is sending and receiving. This is some of what I heard during a two-week period in 1992:

A radio commercial with the slogan "Everything Goes Better with Beer."
The sound of a beer can being opened at 10:00 A.M. on the golf course during a fundraising tournament.
A woman telling the story of her son who attended a prestigious university in the East where, during his first year, he became addicted to drugs and had to be institutionalized. During orientation, parents had been told they needed to "let go" because their children were now adults. However, after her son became addicted, this parent was encouraged to become a part of his treatment plan and was provided accommodations on the university campus. In one short phone call, her parental role was reinstated.

In 1988, an anonymous author wrote the article "To Help Substance Abusers, We Must First Help Ourselves." In his closing paragraph he argued, "When teachers and administrators examine their own thinking and actions to discover attitudes and behaviors that impede progress in this critically important area, schools will become healthier places for everyone. Our students, our society, and ourselves deserve nothing less" (Anonymous, 1988, p. 26). This book is intended to provide just such a professional opportunity.

Historical Perspectives

Higher education's response to alcohol and other drug use has historically been driven by the nature of the relationship between colleges and universities and their students. This relationship has evolved from *in loco parentis* to a consumer–product relationship with legal implications that recognize the special nature of that relationship.

During the time of *in loco parentis,* institutions of higher education attempted to control the use of alcohol and other drugs through rules, regulations, and disciplinary procedures. Possible sanctions for violating the no-use policy included suspension and termination of the student's enrollment. The dean of students was typically the designated super parent with full authority to say "it's my way or the highway." Although there are some administrators who may still long for those "good old days," most agree that the emphasis on the student as an adult was important to the maturing of higher education in the United States. In fact, at the 1988 National Forum on Alcohol and Other Drug Abuse held in Washington, D.C., a panelist suggested that perhaps a return to *in loco parentis* should be considered. The response from the audience of mostly student affairs administrators was clear: "his idea was rebuffed" (Magner, 1988b, p. A37).

As the relationship between colleges and universities and their students evolved, so did their response to alcohol and other drug use on campus. Colleges and universities adjusted policies first to allow those of legal drinking age to consume alcohol in the privacy of their own rooms, and later to extend this privilege to designated public party areas. In addition, due process rights ensured that student disciplinary cases respected the individual students' rights to confidentiality and a fair hearing.

In light of these changes, it is no surprise that most higher education institutions adopted a "responsible drinking" philosophy. According to Milam and Ketcham (1985, p. 192), colleges and universities were not alone in this approach to alcohol; "the federal government spent millions of dollars promoting the idea that alcohol abuse causes alcoholism and that responsible drinking will prevent it. This 'responsible' drinking campaign cultivated the belief that alcoholism is a symptom of psychological and social problems, rather than a physiological disease." During this period, major breweries were even invited on campuses to be a part of the responsible drinking education campaign. The initially reluctant breweries came to welcome the opportunity to develop a direct relationship with their newest consumers.

The Law

In response to public pressures and an increase in traffic fatalities among young adults, states acted to readjust the legal drinking age to 21. As a result of the change in legal drinking age, responsible drinking became an oxymoron for underage students. Suddenly, institutions of higher education found themselves facing an old nemesis—*in loco parentis*. Gibbs and Szablewicz (1988, p. 104) reported, "Courts in several jurisdictions have found the student–college relationship to be a special one that, either explicitly or implicitly, gives rise to a college's duty to protect students from physical harm. . . . To some observers, this trend in the courts has resembled a return to, or a new form of, *in loco parentis* under which colleges must protect students from physical harm but are not empowered to police and control students' morals." In an effort to preserve the positive aspects of the more mature relationship that had emerged, higher education institutions balanced this new "duty to care" with education campaigns that recognized the rights of students as legal adults.

In concert with the notion of duty to care, case law has broadened the boundaries of dram shop laws and social host liabilities in many states. Forty-six of the fifty states currently have dram shop liability and twenty-seven of fifty states have social host liability as a part of their state statutes. In a 1988 Montana case, *Graham v. Montana State University,* involving injury to a high school student enrolled in a summer program, the court held that the university had a custodial relationship and that this duty to care might even extend to cases where it was reasonable and foreseeable that drinking would occur.

Each state has defined the limits of dram shop and social host liability through both legislative action and case law. One good source of information on individual state laws is Gehring and Geraci's *Alcohol on Campus: A Compendium of the Law and a Guide to Campus Policy.* Administrators are encouraged to research the implications of their state criminal and civil liability statutes related to campus policies on alcohol and other drug incidents.

The federal government has also asserted its influence with new legislation such as the Drug-Free Schools and Communities Act. According to Public Law 101–226 section 1213, "Notwithstanding any other provision of law, no institution of higher education shall be eligible to receive funds or any other form of financial assistance under any Federal program, including participation in any federally funded or guaranteed student loan program, unless it certifies to the Secretary that it has adopted and implemented a program to prevent the use of illicit drugs and the abuse of alcohol by students and employees" (The Drug-Free Schools and Communities Act Amendment of 1989). This law clearly requires public institutions to develop drug prevention services or jeopardize their financial aid support for students, as well as any federally funded grants. In addition, the "Student Right to Know" act has required institutions of higher education to disseminate all campus crime information, including information on alcohol and other drug crimes.

No formal identifying term has been agreed upon to describe this new relationship between students and institutions of higher education. However, it appears to be a combination of *in loco parentis,* consumerism, and recognition of the traditional college-aged student as an emerging adult. The legal implications of this relationship represent only one aspect of our institutional responsibility. The public trust placed in educational leaders demands an even more comprehensive view of risk factors that influence student use of illicit drugs and abuse of alcohol.

Students at Risk

The negative consequences of illicit drug use and alcohol abuse are numerous; alcohol-related accidents, accidental overdose of drugs, campus violence including rape and suicide, and greater risk of contracting debilitating diseases such as AIDS and hepatitis B are among the most serious. However, many of the consequences are less visible: poor academic performance, academic withdrawals, residence hall vandalism, relationship problems, and violations of laws. Some populations of students are at greater risk than others of abuse. These high-risk students must be targeted for education and intervention services as a complement to campuswide efforts.

Traditional-Age College Students. Traditional-age college students (ages eighteen to twenty-two) are at greater risk of drug use and alcohol abuse, in part due to the maturation process. As stated by Gonzalez, "in general, the influence of social context (peers, family, and environment) among youth has been more powerful than personality correlates in predicting the initiation of and involvement in problem drinking and other drug usage patterns" (Rivinus, 1988, p. 100).

Perhaps even more important to those who have advocated a developmental approach to working with traditional-age college students is the impact of drinking on the maturation process. According to Gonzales, "The central difficulty for the young adult abuser is the way that the chemical use both interferes with and confuses the normal developmental process" (Rivinus, 1988, p. 150). Despite the retarding effects of alcohol and other drugs on the maturation process, alcohol is the most widely used social rite of passage for traditional-aged students into the culture of higher education. The irony of this rite is its direct and immediate negative impact on the higher-level intellectual functioning that students are seeking through enrollment in higher education.

Students entering higher education are expected to demonstrate their intellectual competence without regard for the difficulty of their life transition. Perhaps this lack of safe passage into the competitive world of academia is one of the underlying influences on the selection of alcohol for peer-to-peer initiation ceremonies. Butler, in his 1993 article, "Alcohol Use by College Students: A Rites of Passage Ritual," presented the following invitation to administrators: "Our challenge, based on an understanding of the importance of rites of passage, is to help current students find or devise rigorous and meaningful rituals that will permit new students to demonstrate their worthiness as members of new groups or subgroups without resorting to dangerous, addictive, and permanently debilitating rituals such as the use and abuse of alcohol" (Butler, 1993, p. 54).

Adult Children of Alcoholics. For students who are adult children of alcoholics (ACOA), the risks of these rituals are far greater. They have already been negatively affected by their family environment in ways that may hamper their pursuit of advanced educational goals. These students are genetically at risk of developing alcoholism as a disease and emotionally at risk in their relationships with others. The potential number of young adults affected by family alcoholism is alarming. "Collegiate children of alcoholics may make up as much as one-third of our student population" (Rivinus, 1988, p. 205). The current movement to integrate ACOA groups onto the college campus is critical in responding to the individual context within which students learn.

Drug-Addicted Students. Students who arrive on the college campus already drug-addicted are obviously at a much higher risk of continued problems. It is important to understand that first use of alcohol typically occurs long before college attendance, even for the traditional-age college student. "Since the average age of a first drink for boys is 11.9 years and for girls is 12.7 years (Rogers, Harris, and Jarmuskewicz, 1987) it is possible to see college-aged alcoholics with drinking histories of ten years or more of regular drinking" (Rivinus, 1988, p. 31). One twenty-year-old student attending Northern

Arizona University told her story this way: "If there ever was a success story, I am the lucky person with it. Five years ago, I was in love with a variety of narcotics. My friends changed, my grades plummeted downward, my self worth was about the true value of the U.S. dollar. The only good thing going for me was my best friend to this day, my mother. . . . I've been sober 5 years . . . and am a campus leader. . . . I plan to use this . . . eventually in a college student related administrative position" (Anonymous, 1993). It is estimated that although only 10 percent or less of the student population might be addicted, many students suffer serious consequences such as accidents or suicide from isolated incidents of intoxication (Rivinus, 1988).

Women. It has been increasingly evident in the research that the use of drugs and alcohol has increased among college women. According to a study released in June 1994, more college women are "drinking to get drunk." The Commission on Substance abuse at colleges and universities found that drinking for the purpose of intoxication among women has more than tripled from 1977 to 1993 (American Council on Education, 1994, p. 7).

The commission's findings are particularly significant because women metabolize alcohol differently from men, and as a result are at higher risk of damaging effects, both immediate and long-term. It is critically important that additional warnings on the effects of alcohol on women be included in prevention messages. Three factors that influence alcohol's increased effect on women have appeared in the literature. These were recently repeated by Hunnicutt, in an article that appeared in *Health News*, as including hormonal influences, the amount of body water, and dehydrogenating effects of alcohol. Hunnicutt warned that "women suffer greater deterioration in abilities to drive and perform other tasks, making them more likely to experience impairment-related consequences" (Hunnicutt, 1994, p. 4). In addition, it has been known for some time that women are more susceptible to breast cancer and cirrhosis of the liver at lower doses and shorter durations than men.

Sexually Active Students. Another area of critical concern on college campuses today is the injurious effect of drug-impaired judgement on sexual activity. Sexual assault and the spread of sexually transmitted diseases, including AIDS, can be both criminal and deadly. "One study found that over 45 percent of students reported being sexually active after drinking or drug use when they might not otherwise have so desired. Over 20 percent engaged in unprotected intercourse while under the influence of drugs (Bloch and Ungerleider, 1986)" (Rivinus, 1988, p. 4). In a more recent survey conducted in April 1992 at Lynchburg College, "41 percent of students said that after drinking they had engaged in sexual activity without using condoms or the precautions they normally would use" (U.S. Center for Substance Abuse Prevention, 1993, p. 4). Furthermore, according to Crichton, the national data on acquaintance rape suggest that "[i]n up to 70 percent of acquaintance rapes, alcohol plays a role" (Crichton, 1993, p. 54). In other words, sex education, though important, is of little use to an impaired student.

Other At-Risk Students. The litany of identified at-risk students is growing longer each year. These students include students from certain ethnic backgrounds (such as Irish), Hispanic males, children of women who drank while pregnant, and children of alcoholics (Metzger, 1988). Rivinius (1988) also includes Native Americans, medical students, the aged, competitive athletes, and anorexic students. Collectively, the population at risk for alcohol and other drug abuse is probably well over 50 percent of the student population, not including those who are the victims of abusers. According to a survey of more than 3,000 college students conducted by Engs and Hanson in 1987–1988, alcohol "was a factor in more than half of the incidents that resulted in physical injury, violent behavior, violation of campus policies, and damage to dormitories and other campus buildings" (Magner, 1988a, p. A37).

Conclusion

The presumption of one right answer has disappeared. Typical college students belong to one or more subcultures that influence their perception and learning process. This is true not only for alcohol and other drug abuse programs, but for all of the typical services provided by student affairs professionals. Alcohol and other drug abuse is not one problem, it is many problems. It does not require one right answer, but many right answers. In order to match services to students we must understand not only the variety of experiences that students bring to the campus, but also the context in which we deliver those services.

The environmental context for developing prevention services includes a full range of institutional types: small liberal arts colleges, community colleges, residential campuses, and large research universities. Each of these communities must match their programs and services to the students enrolled on their campuses. This volume presents information from the largest existing data base on college student alcohol and other drug usage, and suggests multiple right answers for addressing the identified problems.

Higher education did not create alcohol and other drug problems. Alcohol is an integral part of United States' culture and to minimize the negative consequences of its use, prevention programs must be integrated into the fabric of our campus environment. The problem is larger than colleges and universities, and requires collaboration between institutions of higher education and the communities in which they are located. Higher education has an opportunity and responsibility to provide a model of cooperation in response to one of our most difficult social problems. In the final analysis, the possibility exists for the development of new adult relationships with students based on their characteristics and risk status. Nevertheless, there are many bureaucrats who will look for someone to blame, and colleges and universities could easily become the ghost of NOT ME. Those of us in student affairs would be wise to reflect on this Zen master's story.

Circumstances arose one day which delayed preparation of the dinner of a Soto Zen master, Fugai, and his followers. In haste the cook went to the garden with his curved knife and cut off the tops of green vegetables, chopped them together, and made soup, unaware that in his haste he had included a part of a snake in the vegetables.

The followers of Fugai thought they never had tasted such good soup. But when the master himself found the snake's head in his bowl, he summoned the cook. "What is this?" he demanded, holding up the head of the snake.

"Oh, thank you, master," replied the cook, taking the morsel and eating it quickly [Reps, p. 61].

Many colleges and universities have been delayed in preparing effective alcohol and other drug prevention programs on their campuses due to the lack of available information and necessary funding. This book describes efforts occurring today to disseminate information on successful drug prevention programs. But if, in the haste to make up for lost time, student affairs staff accidentally include the head of the snake while preparing an excellent education, it may be best to eat the blame. Let us thank those who criticize. Bow gracefully and quickly swallow our mistakes. There is no time to argue, only to act.

References

Anderson, J., and Binstein, M. "Stopping 'Cat' in Michigan." *Arizona Daily Sun*, October 23, 1993, 48 (68), 6.

Anonymous. "To Help Substance Abusers, We Must First Help Ourselves." *Educational Leadership*, 1988, 45 (6), 20–26.

Anonymous. Personal submission to author. Flagstaff, Ariz., October 1993.

Astin, A. *Preventing Students from Dropping Out*. San Francisco: Jossey-Bass, 1975.

Astin, A. *What Matters in College?: Four Critical Years Revisited*. San Francisco: Jossey-Bass 1992.

Bloch, S. A., and Ungerleider, S. *The Brown University Chemical Dependency Project*. Eugene, Ore.: Integrated Research Services, 1986, pp. 29–65.

Butler, E. "Alcohol Use by College Students: A Rites of Passage Ritual." *NASPA Journal*, 1993, 31 (1), 48–55.

Crichton, S. "Sexual Correctness: Has it Gone Too Far?" *Newsweek*, Oct. 25, 1993, 122, 52–56.

Donovan, B. "Chemical Dependency, Denial, and the Academic Lifestyle." *ACADEME*, 1990, 76 (1), 20–24.

Drug-Free Schools and Communities Act Amendment of 1989. Public Law 101–226, Section 1213.

Feldman, C. "Top Teens Careless: Survey." *Arizona Daily Sun*, October 20, 1993, 48 (65), 1.

Gehring, D. D., and Geraci, C. P. *Alcohol on Campus: A Compendium of the Law and a Guide to Campus Policy*. Asheville, N.C.: College Administration Publications, Inc., 1989.

Gibbs, A., and Szablewicz, J. "Colleges' New Liabilities: An Emerging New In Loco Parentis." *Journal of College Student Development*, March 1988, 29, 104.

Gonzales, G. M., and Broughton, E. "A Status of Alcohol Policies on Campus: A National Survey." *NASPA Journal*, 1986, 24 (2), 49.

Hunnicutt, D. M. "Alcohol Abuse Could Have More Serious Short- and Long-Term Consequences for Women, Researchers Say." *Health News*, 1994, 1 (2), 4.

Johnston, L. D., O'Malley, P. M., and Bachman, J. G. *Drug Use, Drinking, and Smoking: National Survey Results from High School, College, and Young Adults Populations 1975–1988*. Rockville, Md.: National Institute on Drug Abuse, U.S. Department of Health and Human Services, 1989, p. 15.

Johnston, L. D., O'Malley, P. M., and Bachman, J. G. "National Survey Results on Drug Use." *The Monitoring the Future Study, 1975–1992 Volume II. College Students and Young Adults*. National Institute on Drug Abuse Publication no. 93–3598. Rockville, Md.: National Institute on Drug Abuse, 1993.

Kuh, G., and Arnold, J. "Liquid Boarding: A Cultural Analysis of the Role of Alcohol in Fraternity Pledging." *Journal of College Student Development*, Sept. 1993, *34*, 327–334.

Magner, D. "Alcohol-Related Problems Have Not Decreased on Most College Campuses, Survey Indicates." *The Chronicle of Higher Education*, Nov. 9, 1988a, pp. A35 and A37.

Magner, D. "'What Works' in Fighting Drug Abuse." *The Chronicle of Higher Education*, Nov. 9, 1988b, p. A37.

Metzger, L. *From Denial to Recovery: Counseling Problem Drinkers, Alcoholics, and Their Families*. San Francisco: Jossey-Bass, 1988.

Milam, J. R., and Ketcham, K. *Under the Influence: A Guide to the Myths and Realities of Alcoholism*. New York: Bantam Books, 1985.

NCAA. "Ergogenic Drug Use Down; 'Binge-Drinking' on the Rise, According to National Study." *Education Newsletter, NCAA Sports Sciences: An Editorial Supplement to the NCAA News*, Winter 1993.

"Quotable." *The Chronicle of Higher Education*, March 3, 1993, p. B5.

Reps, P. *Zen Flesh, Zen Bones*. New York: Anchor Books, Doubleday, p. 61.

Rivinus, T. M. *Alcoholism/Chemical Dependency and the College Student*. New York: Haworth, 1988.

Rogers, P. D., Harris, J., and Jarmuskewicz, J. *Alcohol and Adolescence. Pediatric Clinics of North America*, 1987, *34* (2), 289–303.

University of Michigan. Press release, January 31, 1994, Ann Arbor: University of Michigan, pp. 1, 3.

U.S. Center for Substance Abuse Prevention. *Put on the Brakes Bulletin*. U.S. Department of Health and Human Services, March 1993, p. 4.

Wertz, R. (ed.). "Our Children at Risk." *The Chemical People Newsletter*, Sept.–Oct. 1991.

EILEEN V. COUGHLIN is vice president for student affairs/dean for academic support services at Western Washington University, Bellingham. She was also director of the qualitative evaluation project presented in chapters Six and Seven.

In order to better understand the magnitude and consequences of alcohol abuse and other drug use, myths must be confronted with facts. Student affairs administrators are well positioned to expose the fantasy surrounding these myths.

Facts and Myths

Cheryl A. Presley, Philip W. Meilman, Julie F. Padgett

Myths have extraordinary power. They are perceptions passed on to others as facts and are often embedded with rules of behavior and instructions about handling the complexities of life. A few examples are "men like women to drink with them," or "beer and masculinity go hand in hand," and perhaps the most common perception acted out on America's college campuses, "drinking is an important part of college life." To develop successful alcohol prevention programs on college campuses, administrators must examine these myths and determine whether they are factually correct. The need for factually correct information is highlighted by Mark Harrison Moore. In an article in *The Chronicle of Higher Education* he writes, "We need to study just how norms of drug-related behavior emerge and operate in society. For example, we do not yet know whether behavior can be influenced by education programs, laws, or propaganda campaigns. Nor do we know under what circumstances those efforts produce a backlash. Since much of drug policy is concerned with shaping citizens' attitudes and actions, our lack of knowledge is crippling" (Moore, 1989, p. 56). Faculty, students, parents, and alumni look to student services administrators to provide perspectives on campus problems and to offer specific solutions to those problems. To identify possible solutions, administrators must first separate myths from facts regarding alcohol use on their campuses.

The intent of this chapter is to dispel myths with facts about alcohol abuse and other drug use on America's college campuses. The six myths addressed were identified from a national survey of 58,000 college students. Additionally, specific suggestions are made for student services administrators with strategies for addressing the culture surrounding alcohol abuse and other drug use and methods for educating all constituencies.

One of the most significant myths that dramatically affects use on college campuses is the myth that alcohol is predominantly a sedative or depressant drug. In *Under the Influence,* Milam and Ketcham (1985) point out that alcohol, when used in small amounts, directly stimulates nerve tissues. After one or two drinks, the drinker feels happy, talkative, energetic, and even euphoric. The drinker may also experience some improvement in thought and performance. However, as an individual's blood alcohol level rises, the amount of alcohol in the brain increases and begins to disturb the brain's electrical and chemical circuitry. As the brain begins to malfunction, behavior changes such as slurred speech and an unsteady gait become obvious as alcohol is transformed into a depressant or sedative. At this point, drinking behavior can result in a variety of negative consequences to the college student.

This fact is responsible for producing the campus life issue of greatest concern. If it were not for the initially stimulating effects of alcohol, many people would lose interest in drinking. As alcohol's sedative effects begin to take over and dysphoria begins to predominate, the pleasure and excitement of drinking are gradually canceled out. If alcohol acted only as a depressant, possibly alcohol use would no longer be a primary concern for student services administrators. Thus, combatting the myth that alcohol acts only as a depressant is a major challenge of the 1990s for student services administrators on American college campuses.

The value in understanding myths is evident in the potential impact of problem drinking. Kinney and Leaton (Sherwood, 1987) estimated that for every problem drinker, at least four other people are negatively affected. Using this conservative number, one can calculate the potential impact on the campus. The numbers identify a significant need for student services administrators to first assess alcohol use on their campus and then to respond to the problem by communicating their findings to all constituencies. Through this educational process, the tone and culture of alcohol and other drug use can be better understood and subsequently altered.

In an effort to assess college students' alcohol and other drug use, an instrument was developed in 1989 by a group supported by the 1987 Fund for the Improvement of Postsecondary Education (FIPSE)-funded drug prevention programs. The committee was initially charged with selecting a survey tool for assessing alcohol and other drug use on campuses. The committee quickly discovered that none of the existing questionnaires adequately addressed their needs. To fill the void, the committee developed the Core Alcohol and Drug Survey, so named because it was to be the centerpiece or "core" around which campuses could ask other questions specific to their institutions. At the same time, the core questions would ensure that institutions asked the same questions in the same way to establish normative data and allow for statistical comparisons with those norms.

The Core Alcohol and Drug Survey is a single-page, two-sided, machine-scored questionnaire that includes items on demographics, alcohol and drug use frequency, age of first use, perceptions of students' use and campus policy, family history, and consequences of use. It takes approximately fifteen minutes for students to complete, and an institution's data can be analyzed and returned within ten days of submission to the scoring center. The institution is provided with its own report, and the raw data, stripped of institutional identification, are aggregated with data from other schools, thereby creating a national data base. In the first year of its publication, seventy-eight institutions of higher education used the Core Alcohol and Drug Survey. This yielded data on more than 58,000 students. The demographic composition of the students in this data base approximated the characteristics gathered by the National Center for Educational Statistics for that year with respect to gender, race, and year in school. From these data, two important publications have appeared to date, including a short report to college presidents and a more detailed monograph that provides data for each of the questions on the survey (Presley and Meilman, 1992; Presley, Meilman, and Lyerla, 1993).

In the material that follows, data from the Core national data base is used to examine six common beliefs and to determine whether they are myth or fact.

Belief One: The consequences of college drinking and drug use are minimal; students mostly experience just headaches or hangovers.

There are a substantial number of consequences that students report experiencing, some of which are headaches and hangovers. However, there are far more extensive consequences. As shown in Table 2.1, the percentage of students

Table 2.1. Consequence in the Last Year of Alcohol and Other Drug Use by Age of Students

	Percentage of Students Experiencing Consequence at Least Once in Past Year	
Consequence	Under 21	Over 21
Hangover	65.9%	59.1%
Hangover more than five times	23.4	19.6
Poor academic performance	26.6	19.5
Trouble with authorities	17.7	8.5
Vandalism	9.8	5.3
Arguments or fights	38.8	19.5
Nausea or vomiting	57.0	41.6
Driving while intoxicated	34.9	36.6
Missed classes	32.7	26.1
Criticism for substance abuse	50.3	22.5
Thought I might have a problem	11.7	11.8
Memory loss	33.1	22.2
Done something I regretted	45.4	32.1
Arrests for DWI, DUI	1.4	2.0
Sexual misconduct	18.4	11.0
Unsuccessful attempt to stop using	6.2	5.4
Suicide attempt or thoughts	6.6	4.3
Injury	20.7	10.7

Note: N = 55,670; under 21 = 29,997; 21 or older = 25,673.

both above and below the legal drinking age who reported experiencing various negative consequences within the twelve-month period before they filled out the Core Alcohol and Drug Survey is noteworthy, as are the differences between the age groups.

As can be seen, 38.8 percent of the students under the age of twenty-one reported they had been in an argument or a fight due to alcohol or other drug use, 50.3 percent had been criticized for substance abuse, and almost 20.7 percent reported being hurt or injured during the previous year. These consequences occurred in underage students at rates almost double those of students twenty-one and over.

Many of the negative consequences that students reported experiencing include those that affect academic performance. Combining the data for all students reveals that 28 percent had a memory loss, 30 percent missed class, and 23 percent performed poorly on a test or other important project. In addition, we found that heavier alcohol consumption is associated with lower GPAs, as shown in Figure 2.1.

Although these numbers speak directly about the potential impact on retention, performance, and behaviors of students, they are still numerical abstractions that may be easily dismissed unless one looks at human factors. The following statements by students about drinking and their grades provide a more personal interpretation of the data.

> I go to a junior college now. I was put on probation because I partied too much. I kept dropping classes until I couldn't drop anymore.

> I dropped out of school two years ago because I drank too much. I didn't recognize I was partying too much. I would wake up with hangovers every morning and my GPA kept falling. I realized then that I needed to take a look at my behavior.

Issues surrounding drinking "too much" appear to concern many college students. There appears to be something of an imperative to be a part of the drinking culture, but the rules are confusing and often contradictory.

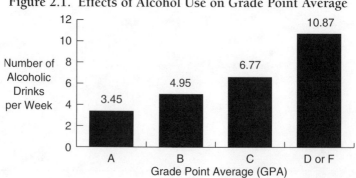

Figure 2.1. Effects of Alcohol Use on Grade Point Average

I think that there is no middle—either you have to be pro getting wasted or pro not using at all. I don't know what responsible drinking is.

Belief Two: Drinking and getting rip-roaring drunk are important parts of college life. After all, these are the best years of your life.

I was at a party on another campus and had half a bottle of rum, half a bottle of gin, and who knows what else before I passed out. I woke up, puked, then passed out several times throughout the night. Other than that, I can't remember anything at all.

I saw a friend throwing up all over himself and get laughed at. Then he still wanted more.

One night on the way to a party, I saw a girl walking home by herself stone drunk. She couldn't even stay on the sidewalk. Anything could have happened.

Overall, the Core Alcohol and Drug Survey showed that 42 percent of the students surveyed reported having binged on alcohol in the previous two weeks, as can be seen in Table 2.2. Binge drinking is operationally defined as the consumption of five or more drinks in one sitting. These data are consistent with findings from some earlier studies. Wechsler and Isaac (1992) found that 42 percent of first-year students in Massachusetts had engaged in binge drinking in the previous two weeks. Johnston, O'Malley, and Bachman (1991) reported that the proportion of binge drinkers in their national college sample varied between 41 percent and 45 percent during the years from 1980 to 1990.

The Core Survey data show that 28 percent of the students reported having binged two or more times in the previous fourteen days. A substantially greater percentage of students under the legal drinking age (48 percent) engaged in binge drinking during the previous two weeks than students who

Table 2.2. Frequency of Binge Drinking Episodes in the Previous Two Weeks

	Percentage of Students		
Number of Episodes	Male	Female	Total
None	48.6%	65.0%	58.2%
One	13.7	13.6	13.7
Two	10.9	8.6	9.6
3 to 5	16.2	9.2	12.1
6 to 9	6.6	2.3	4.1
10 or more	3.8	1.3	2.3

Note: N = 53,299; male = 22,135; female = 31,164.

were twenty-one and older (35 percent). Binge drinking is frequently associ-ated with sexual assault, fights, drunken driving, and property damage, and so these findings are of particular concern to those who work in student services.

Binge drinking by students residing in fraternity or sorority houses is especially concerning, for it occurs frequently and is not confined to week-ends. Data from the Core Alcohol and Drug Survey indicate that 74 percent of Greek house residents reported episodes of binge drinking in the previous two weeks, compared with 42 percent for all students. Furthermore, 22 per-cent of Greek house residents reported bingeing more than five times in the previous two weeks as compared with 6 percent of all students, Greek and non-Greek. Seven percent of Greek house residents reported binge drinking almost every night.

Alarming case reports about drinking occur each year on virtually every college campus in the nation, and these reports add depth to the statistics. One such report was that of a student who reported that he had been drinking heavily with the encouragement of his friends. Having lost count of the num-ber of drinks that he had consumed, he suffered a blackout and was found out-side his residence hall, passed out beneath the bushes. Fortunately, someone found him a few hours later and called an ambulance. This student had a blood alcohol concentration (BAC) of 0.32 percent, a near lethal dose for those without high tolerance. More alarming, he had experienced hypothermia on his hands and feet that resulted in a permanent loss of feeling in his fingers—this despite the fact that it was August and 90 degrees outside.

On another campus, a student who chugged alcohol was taken to the emergency room with a BAC of 0.47 percent. He was unresponsive and placed on life support. An hour later, his BAC was measured at 0.49 percent. The student spent several days in intensive care, developed pneumonia, took the rest of the semester off, and was left with a medical bill in the thousands of dollars.

Stories like these are becoming all too common on our campuses. The asso-ciated myths that student drinking is not harmful, that partying is harmless fun, and that "boys will be boys" may be most harmful. Assurances that serious consequences affect only a few students do not necessarily reflect the reality. The best years of your life may be altogether lost in the college drinking culture.

Belief Three: Women drink less than men, so there is less need to target them in programming efforts.

It is true that fewer female students binge drink than males, but still 35 per-cent of the women taking the Core Alcohol and Drug Survey reported binge drinking episodes in the previous two weeks. In addition, the prevalence of reported alcohol use in the last year is no different for females than for males

(85 percent). Also of concern is the fact that women living in Greek houses reported drinking twice as much alcohol as female students as a whole, six drinks per week as opposed to three drinks. (For men, the figures were 20.3 drinks per week for fraternity house residents and 7.5 drinks for all male students.) These findings about women's drinking patterns conflict with the perception that women are not at risk for alcohol-related problems.

Women, in general, reported somewhat fewer consequences as a result of alcohol or other drug use than men, but the numbers are still significant. As shown in Table 2.3, three-fifths of the women surveyed reported hangovers in the previous year, and more than a quarter of them suffered blackouts. It has been documented that women who drink regularly have special health concerns. They are more prone to breast cancer and, if pregnant, risk causing fetal alcohol syndrome in their children. Perhaps even more importantly, according to Lawson and Lawson (1989, pp. 14–15), "Women become intoxicated more easily than men on the same amount of alcohol even if they weigh the same because women generally have less muscle tissue, which contains the water to break down the alcohol. . . . Women may develop cirrhosis of the liver at lower levels of alcohol consumption and after a shorter history of excessive drinking than do men."

Sexual victimization and acquaintance rape under the influence are particularly alarming and have received a good deal of national publicity. Surveys and research studies have clearly demonstrated a connection between alcohol and sexual activity (Butcher, Manning, and O'Neal, 1991; Koss and

Table 2.3. **Percentage of Men and Women Students Reporting Various Consequences of Alcohol and Other Drug Use**

Consequence	Male	Female
Hangover	66.9%	59.9%
Poor academic performance	27.7	20.3
Trouble with authorities	19.9	9.0
Vandalism	14.3	3.1
Arguments or fights	35.3	31.9
Nausea or vomiting	51.7	48.9
Driving under the influence	43.1	30.4
Arrests for DWI, DUI	3.0	0.7
Missed classes	35.5	26.4
Criticism for substance abuse	33.1	26.2
Thought I might have a problem	16.1	8.6
Memory loss	29.9	26.9
Done something I regretted	41.5	37.8
Sexual misconduct	14.7	15.2
Unsuccessful attempt to stop using	7.8	4.3
Suicide attempt or thoughts	5.4	5.6
Injury	18.9	14.2

Note: N = 51,971; males = 21,458; females = 30,513.

Dinero, 1989; Meilman, 1993; Miller and Marshall, 1987; Muehlenhard and Linton, 1987), but comments made by students themselves tell the story more graphically:

> The girl had way too much to drink and was wandering off randomly; we had trouble keeping up with her. She disappeared and could not be found. The next morning she woke up in some strange room of a guy and could not remember what had happened the past night.

> A girl who gets drunk a lot is thought of as a slut even if she doesn't hook up with someone.

> Went to a date party. My date took me upstairs to drink before the party. I drank too much because I was nervous. Later, I did some things I didn't want to because I was drunk and I felt I had to.

Clearly, there is as much need to target women in prevention programming as there is to target men. We need to teach both men and women the meaning of respect and responsibility in relationships, and we need to emphasize the need to make decisions about sexual activity before taking the first drink.

Belief Four: Everyone drinks to excess.

Although 85 percent of the students reported using alcohol in the last year, approximately 33 percent reported that they preferred to live in an alcohol-free environment and 87 percent preferred a drug-free environment. Furthermore, more than half the students said that they consumed one or fewer drinks per week, on average. Looking at the 58 percent of students who did not report binge drinking in the previous two weeks, the differences in preferences for an alcohol- and drug-free environment become even more pronounced; 64 percent of the nonbingers preferred an alcohol-free environment and 93 percent of them preferred a drug-free environment. These findings contrast with the widely held perception that all students want to drink and drink to excess.

Perkins and Berkowitz (1986) have shown that perceptions of alcohol use on campus are greater than the actual usage levels, leading students to believe they should drink to the level of the perception in order to fit in. In other words, if students believe or perceive that other students binge drink, they will adjust their consumption level to meet that perception. Implied in this is the idea that they can also lower their consumption if the perceptions are corrected. Given that the Core Alcohol and Drug Survey reflects a significant number of students who want to live in a substance-free environment, it is conceivable that drinking levels would drop if the information showing lower usage levels is disseminated. Such an education program was attempted at Northern Illinois University and there was a corresponding drop in the level of binge drinking (Haines, 1992). This may be a fruitful area for further exploration.

Student assumptions regarding alcohol and other drug use and the message students give each other are part of the culture that keeps alcohol and other drug use firmly in place despite the fact that so many students say they would prefer a substance-free environment. We need to give these students a voice.

Belief Five: There are certain locations where students can go to college that will shield them from alcohol and other drug abuse.

The reality is that alcohol continues to be the most frequently used drug for college students regardless of age, institutional characteristics, or region. However, there do appear to be some regional differences in the average number of drinks consumed per week. As Figure 2.2 indicates, the Northeast showed a consumption level more than double that of the West. The North Central region had the second highest consumption level, and the South ranked third. Consistent with these findings, the West and the South had the lowest percentage of students reporting binge drinking episodes and the Northeast had the highest.

Figure 2.2. Average Number of Drinks per Week and Percent Bingeing in the Previous Two Weeks

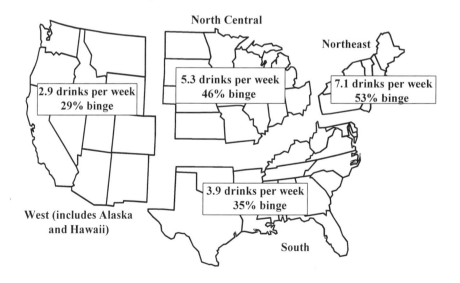

North Central

Northeast

2.9 drinks per week
29% binge

5.3 drinks per week
46% binge

7.1 drinks per week
53% binge

3.9 drinks per week
35% binge

West (includes Alaska and Hawaii)

South

There is significant concern regarding the use of drugs other than alcohol. Table 2.4 presents the annual prevalence figures for the most frequently used drugs among students at institutions of higher education by region of the country. As can be seen, no region is exempt from illicit drug use. Overall, approximately 26 percent of the students reported using marijuana in the previous twelve months and 5 percent reported using cocaine, using hallucinogens, and using amphetamines.

At the same time, some differences emerged when we examined alcohol consumption data by institutional size. As shown in Table 2.5, average weekly alcohol consumption was inversely proportional to the size of the institution, particularly for men's drinking. This contradicts the assumption that there is less alcohol abuse at small schools that provide more individualized attention for students.

Belief Six: There is little that can be done to change things.

This volume is dedicated to showing what works. As we search for answers to the drug and alcohol problems on campus, it is essential to remember that large-scale change is the product of many small changes. Altering habits, perceptions, and norms is a challenge that requires clear vision, small changes, and persistence.

By examining our longitudinal data, we found that campuses with FIPSE-funded drug prevention programs showed modest reductions in alcohol and

Table 2.4. Prevalence of the Most Frequently Used Drugs in the Previous Year by Region

Region	Tobacco	Marijuana	Cocaine	Hallucinogens	Amphetamines
West	31.4	23.2	6.5	3.9	4.1
North Central	42.4	23.4	3.8	3.8	5.1
South	39.0	22.2	4.6	5.3	6.0
Northeast	45.5	37.3	6.3	7.3	4.8

Note: N = 56,244.

Table 2.5. Average Number of Drinks per Week by Size of Institution

	Average Number of Drinks per Week		
Size of institution	Male	Female	Total
Less than 2,500	10.2	4.3	6.6
2,500 to 4,999	7.5	2.7	4.7
5,000 to 9,999	7.5	3.1	4.9
10,000 to 19,999	6.9	3.0	4.7
20,000 or more	4.7	2.0	3.2

Note: N = 53,143; male = 22,133; female = 31,010.

other drug use from 1990 to 1991. In the 37 campuses that conducted pre- and post-assessments of their drug prevention programs, there was a decrease in the average number of drinks consumed per week from 4.95 drinks to 4.80 drinks. (Although this change may seem small, it is important to consider that these figures are averaged across tens of thousands of students.) Correspondingly, there was an increase in the number of students who reported an absence of binge drinking in the previous two weeks, with the percentage of non-bingers rising from 56 percent to 60 percent. There was also a modest reduction in the percentage of students reporting negative consequences from alcohol and other drug use.

Students are a greater resource than they are often thought to be. However, to date, only 7 percent of the 58,000 students surveyed reported that they were actively involved in drug prevention programming efforts. Clearly, we have not tapped this large resource for change as much as we could.

The question remains to be answered, What types of programs work? What activities have the greatest effect on campus culture to promote a drug-free environment? As the answers to these questions unfold, it is evident that the best natural resources we have may be the students themselves.

Administrative Action

Detaching myth from reality is a significant challenge. As evidenced in the research results reported in this chapter, many college students live their lives as if the myths of alcohol use and abuse are reality. Because myths can be dispelled with facts, the following suggestions are made to help administrators begin to dispel the prevailing myths.

Administration

Assess faculty and administrators' attitudes toward alcohol use. This allows student services administrators to assess the culture of the institution as it relates to alcohol use and provides an opportunity to identify the tone and environment of the institution.

Assess the example you set for faculty, students, and administrators regarding alcohol use. Does your behavior support or negate the campus alcohol policy?

Assess the effectiveness of existing alcohol and drug prevention programs on campus. One characteristic of success, described in Chapter Six of this volume, is support from the top administrative levels. To assess your current programs, use the self-assessment tool included in Chapter Seven.

Education

Disseminate statistical data from the Core instrument relating to social, medical, and especially academic consequences to incoming students, parents, alumni, faculty, and other administrators. For example, data from Belief One substantiate that the number of drinks consumed per week directly correlates with students' grade point averages. Data from Belief Three provide information about negative consequences that are also persistence issues (such as poor academic performance, missed classes, and memory loss resulting from alcohol and other drug use).

Communicate clearly to alumni and administrators about the ethical obligations to serve as role models for the current student population. Pay particular attention to alumni who were previously involved in Greek organizations.

Communicate the alcohol policy clearly and frequently to the student body. It is important to reiterate the policy each year.

Deliver consistent responses to violations of policy, including education along with sanctions.

In summary, student services administrators are responsible for assessing alcohol and drug use on their campuses, understanding the tone and culture of various constituencies across campus, and giving voice to factual realities in order to correct myths relating to alcohol use. This charge goes far beyond the historical emphasis on targeting the 10 percent estimated to demonstrate addictive behaviors. The vast numbers of students affected by use and abuse and the need to move to a wellness approach must be addressed through effective programs. It is the hope of the authors that the information gleaned from this publication in combination with the self-assessment tool in Chapter Seven will provide student services administrators with strategies to address the culture surrounding alcohol abuse and other drug use on college and university campuses.

References

Butcher, A. H., Manning, D. T., and O'Neal, E. C. "HIV-Related Sexual Behaviors of College Students." *Journal of American College Health,* 1991, *40* (3), 115–118.

Haines, M. Personal communication. De Kalb: Northern Illinois University, 1992.

Johnston, L. D., O'Malley, P. M., and Bachman, J. G. *Drug Use Among American High School Seniors, College Students, and Young Adults, 1975–1990.* Vol. 2, *College Students and Young Adults.* National Institute on Drug Abuse, U.S. Department of Health and Human Services, Public Health Service, Alcohol, Drug Abuse, and Mental Health Administration, DHHS Publication No. (ADM) 91–1835. Washington, D.C.: Government Printing Office, 1991, p. 143.

Koss, M. P., and Dinero, T. E. "Discriminant Analysis of Risk Factors for Sexual Victimization Among a National Sample of College Women." *Journal of Consulting and Clinical Psychology,* 1989, *57,* 242–250.

Lawson, G. W., and Lawson, A. W. *Alcoholism and Substance Abuse in Special Populations.* Rockville, Md.: Aspen, 1989, pp. 14–15.

Meilman, P. W. "Alcohol-Induced Sexual Behavior on Campus." *Journal of American College Health,* 1993, *42* (1), 27–31.

Milam, J. R., and Ketcham, K. *Under the Influence: A Guide to Myths and Realities of Alcoholism.* New York: Bantam, 1985.

Miller, B., and Marshall, J. C. "Coercive Sex on the University Campus." *Journal of College Student Personnel,* 1987, *28,* 38–47.

Moore, M. H. "Point of View: Academe and Government Must Collaborate to Confront the Drug Crisis." *The Chronicle of Higher Education,* November 29, 1989, p. 56.

Muehlenhard, C. L., Linton, M. A. "Date Rape and Sexual Aggression in Dating Situations: Incidence and Risk Factors." *Journal of Counseling Psychology,* 1987, *34,* 186–196.

Perkins, H. W., and Berkowitz, A. D. "Perceiving the Community Norms of Alcohol Use Among Students: Some Research Implications for Campus Alcohol Education Programming." *International Journal of the Addictions,* 1986, *21* (9/10), 961–976.

Presley, C. A., and Meilman, P. W. *Alcohol and Drugs on American College Campuses: A Report to College Presidents.* Carbondale: Southern Illinois University, 1992.

Presley, C. A., Meilman, P. W., and Lyerla, R. *Alcohol and Drugs on American College Campuses: Use, Consequences, and Perceptions of the Campus Environment, Vol. I: 1989–91.* Carbondale: Southern Illinois University, 1993.

Sherwood, J. S. "Alcohol Policies and Practices on College and University Campuses." *NASPA monograph, Series 7.* National Association of Student Personnel Administrators, July 1987.

Wechsler, H., and Isaac, N. "Binge Drinkers at Massachusetts Colleges: Prevalence, Drinking Style, Time Trends, and Associated Problems." *Journal of the American Medical Association,* June 3, 1992, *267* (21), 2929–2931.

CHERYL A. PRESLEY *is executive director of the Core Institute at Southern Illinois University at Carbondale.*

PHILIP W. MEILMAN *is director of the counseling center and research professor of psychology at the College of William and Mary.*

JULIE F. PADGETT *is associate athletic director at Northern Arizona University.*

*Capturing the attention of college and university presidents
regarding alcohol and other drug use requires an understanding
of their public role and of the relationship of prevention to the
particular mission of your institution. Leaders in student
development must link prevention to their presidents' agendas.*

Hooking Your President on Prevention

Paul C. Gianini, Jr., Ruth L. Nicholson

College and university presidents have the privilege and responsibility of leading their institutions into the next century. Society expects higher education to
instill and inspire the next generation of leaders with an improved set of values to achieve a more positive, productive society. This leadership includes
empowering students, academic faculty, and administrators, and extends into
the community.

No college campus is immune to the problems and consequences of alcohol and drug abuse. One example of these problems is the increase in severity
of discipline issues on campuses throughout the country. The correlation
between these problems and the use of alcohol and other substances is clear.
For years, the use of these substances by college-age students was deemed
appropriate—a rite of passage—and the attitude of college administrators,
including the omnipotent president, was one of benign neglect.

Today, the attitude toward the use of alcohol and illicit drugs has begun
to change as more and more related tragedies threaten the fiber of society. Colleges have had to respond to legislation that raised the legal age to purchase
and consume alcohol. College and university presidents have struggled with
the ethical and moral dilemmas of their role and the responsibility of their
institution in providing leadership in the prevention of alcohol and other drug
abuse. The enforcement of these laws within the context of a more mature
administrator–student relationship presents a dilemma for institutions of
higher education. Administrators must juggle enforcement requirements leg-
islated by local and state drinking laws against developmental educational
approaches that represent a more mature relationship with students.

New Directions for Student Services, no. 67, Fall 1994   © Jossey-Bass Publishers

In addition, despite all the education prevention efforts of the late 1980s, a joint report of the Carnegie Foundation (1990) indicated that alcohol is still a major problem. According to this survey of 382 college and university presidents, "52 percent of the college presidents said the quality of campus life was a greater concern than a few years ago; two-thirds of the presidents considered alcohol abuse a 'moderate' or 'major' problem" (p. 38). Eigen (1991) said it even more directly in his white paper to the U.S. Department of Education: "presidents classified alcohol abuse as the campus life issue of their greatest concern" (p. 1). Too many students have become hooked on alcohol and drugs and, as a result, have lost their educational potential and the resulting contributions to society. College campuses are experiencing a paradigm shift, empowering students, faculty, and administrators to be hooked on prevention, by changing their campus environments.

Presidents' agendas are full of instructional concerns, funding predicaments, and legislative challenges. Today's college and university presidents need to be hooked on the issue of drug and alcohol prevention. Capturing the attention of the president and putting prevention on his or her agenda is a leadership role of deans and directors of student affairs.

To gain the president's attention, it is vital to know what the president will find the most interesting and motivating. Hooking a president on prevention is a dynamic process that infuses prevention into the president's interests and the culture of the institution. Prevention is not a separate agenda issue, but rather an underlying factor in student success.

All college and university presidents share certain roles and interests, be they CEOs of Ivy League universities, four-year institutions, or community colleges. Presidents are concerned about the impact of alcohol and drug abuse on the mission of their institution and on society at large. John Welty, president of California State University, Fresno, in a speech at the 1989 Network Conference expressed the belief of many presidents: "Colleges and universities have long been concerned about the abuse of alcohol and other drugs. The escalating abuse of alcohol and other drugs in society, however, has made it necessary for colleges and universities to take a completely new look at their campus approach to this issue. There is no doubt that the abuse of alcohol and other drugs has disastrous implications for our economic system and quality of life, and thereby poses a serious threat to society." The economic system and quality of life are important agendas for presidents. Alcohol and drug prevention programs provide presidents the opportunity to be part of the solution by linking higher education to the larger community. Their awareness of the changing norms in society and the consequences of alcohol and drug abuse makes it possible for presidents to encourage and nurture the relationship between the campus and the community.

Deans of students and directors of prevention programs are in a leadership position to become the campus experts on federal legislation, comprehensive policies, and effective program models. As experts, they should have the knowledge and skills to provide their presidents with up-to-date information. Prevention tacticians should be aware of the strategies identified by Lofquist (1989, p. 13):

Prevention is realistic and goal-oriented.
Prevention is practical and specific.
Prevention is designed to attain measurable results.
Prevention is focused on short- and long-range impact.
Prevention is cost-effective and cost-reducing.
Prevention is not just a luxury, but a necessity if a balanced community approach to human development is to be achieved.

Prevention strategies are most effective when based on assessment data. Colleges and universities need to have concrete knowledge of the substance abuse problems on their campuses in order to develop appropriate prevention goals and strategies and to measure environmental change. These data provide the basis for program development and evaluation.

Assessment Strategies

Deans and directors of student life, as the institution's prevention tacticians, must determine which survey instruments provide the data that will be most helpful to their colleges in developing successful prevention strategies. Survey results afford presidents the documentation that assesses campus climates. Presidents are interested in the results of surveys and can be extremely sensitive if survey results are presented in a negative manner. However, even if survey results present a negative picture of the institution, connecting them to program outcomes is a proactive approach. Presidents should always be well-briefed before survey results are disseminated to other college offices. Short briefing papers that profile their campus's alcohol and drug behavior and compare their campus to institutions of similar size and type, tied to program goals, provide presidents with the appropriate information.

The Core Alcohol and Drug Survey (Presley, Meilman, and Lyerla, 1993) was intended to be the core or center of assessment that provides higher education institutions a profile of the issues and behaviors on their campuses (see Chapter Two, this volume). The content areas of the Core Survey were designed to provide campus leaders with statistically reliable and valid information about the campus and drug and alcohol climate.

Another instrument, developed by Northern Arizona University, is described in Chapter Six of this volume. Their research found that strong administrative support from the top is an essential factor in effective programs (Mills-Novoa, 1992).

Although many presidents are committed to infusing prevention into their institutions, some institutions are struggling. These struggling institutions need the leadership of a president committed to prevention. Hooking your president on prevention involves developing strategies that make prevention an integral, contributing part of the institution. These strategies should empower the president to be a more effective campus and community leader. The following five strategies have proven successful in gaining the attention and commitment of presidents: link prevention to mission, vision, and culture of institution; develop clear, effective policies; develop a commitment and plan for resource development; develop good press opportunities for your president and institution to be recognized as a leader in prevention; and strengthen the role of the president in the local community.

Mission, Vision, and Culture. There is a synergistic relationship between presidents and the mission, culture, and values of their institution. Prevention programs can become a leading theme of the president and can contribute to the mission of the institution. Judith A. Sturnick, president of Keene State College, challenges the relationship between the president and the mission and values of the institution. "The institutional self definition that only a vision can create becomes more critical in a time of downsizing, resource constraint, and contracting missions. In this climate, we need more than ever to have institutional visions that challenge us internally, while signifying us externally. The president's voice must embody the institutional imperatives of that vision and focus the values of the campus" (1993, p. 5). The president's priorities establish the vision and tone of the institution. Prevention can be a major theme of presidents in implementing their vision. As a part of this vision and tone, the Carnegie Foundation for the Advancement of Teaching, in a special report titled *Campus Life,* suggests six principles for strengthening campus communities:

> First, a college or university is an educationally *purposeful* community, a place where faculty and students share academic goals and work together to strengthen teaching and learning on the campus.
>
> Second, a college or university is an *open* community, a place where freedom of expression is uncompromisingly protected and where civility is powerfully affirmed.
>
> Third, a college or university is a *just* community, a place where the sacredness of the person is honored and where diversity is aggressively pursued.
>
> Fourth, a college or university is a *disciplined* community, a place where individuals accept their obligations to the group and where well-defined governance procedures guide behavior for the common good.
>
> Fifth, a college or university is a *caring* community, a place where the well-being of each member is sensitively supported and where service to others is encouraged.
>
> Sixth, a college or university is a *celebration* community, one in which the heritage of the institution is remembered and where rituals affirming both tradition and change are widely shared. [1990, pp. 7–8]

By integrating these principles into campus life, student services professionals can transform the campus climate. Prevention programs provide their leaders the tools to empower individuals to strengthen the campus community.

By infusing prevention programs throughout the institution, campus leaders can make prevention a vital part of both the academic and student affairs programs. Senge (1990, p. 181) states that "in the learning organization, the new 'dogma' will be vision, values, and mental models." Presidents are symbols of institutions' vision and values. A major role of the president in developing vision is that of strategic planner. Deans and directors of prevention programs should be actively involved in the planning process. Presidents need to know the extent of the substance abuse problems on campus and how prevention programs can prevent future problems. No matter how extensive the problem, helping the president to prevent or correct the problem is a valuable role to both the campus and the community it serves.

Colleges and universities are learning organizations whose mission is to educate and train tomorrow's leaders. Deans and directors of prevention programs need to link campus issues such as student retention and student success to prevention programs such as peer support networks and curriculum infusion. These linkages must have a visible presence in strategic planning documents. Presidents are likely to support efforts that strengthen the mission and values of the institutions and create a more effective learning organization.

Ronald Bucknam, director of the Drug Prevention Program for the Fund for the Improvement of Postsecondary Education (FIPSE), has identified four ways institutions of higher education can develop academic growth and empower the institution to develop a healthier climate:

> First, it can help to bring together the one third of the students who have as a common bond the preference not to have alcohol and other drugs at the parties that they attend on and around campus. Thus, they may begin to know that they are not alone but are part of a large and significant group—a group that agrees on positive behavioral norms regarding campus drug and alcohol use and knows how that use negatively affects the learning and social environment.
>
> Second, it can help empower those students as they seek to implement their own positive norms for campus behavior.
>
> Third, it can plan for a change in the institutional environment that gives students permission to be true to their own positive values and to have those values define the campus cultural scene.
>
> Fourth, the institution's leaders can rethink and revise the internal organization to create opportunities and provide support for the creation and sustenance of the new critical mass, the new cultural scene, and the new behavioral norms. Such a new environment will support students, and staff, and faculty in their quest for positive learning and social interaction and will support the institution in its efforts to provide students with the opportunity for intellectual and social development. [1994, p. 307]

Campuses throughout the country are developing new campus communities by providing options both in student life and student activities such as alcohol-free residence halls and weekend or evening intramural sporting events. Prevention programs that strengthen the vision and values of the institution by creating and supporting a critical mass of students, faculty, and administrators are most likely to find strong support from their president.

Clear, Effective Policy. Colleges and universities have responded to recent legislation by developing policies and procedures. Presidents have looked to their deans and directors for guidance. Taking a strong leadership role in developing policy is vital in gaining the attention and commitment of presidents. Being knowledgeable about state and federal laws and the position national organizations have taken on these laws provides the blueprint for policy development. Presidents rely on their vice presidents, deans, and directors for leadership in developing programs to meet the needs of students and interpret new legislation. In order to ensure the president's success, prevention personnel must be acutely aware of the legislation affecting campus prevention efforts.

Federal legislation affecting alcohol and drug issues in higher education began in 1986, when President Reagan signed into law the Omnibus Anti-Drug Bill that provided a total of $1.66 billion dollars to fund new anti–drug abuse initiatives (The Drug Abuse Report, 1986). This legislation established an active federal role in drug education. The Drug-Free Schools and Communities Act of 1986 contained in that legislation made available $7.6 million in grants to colleges and universities for prevention programs. FIPSE, within the Department of Education, was given the responsibility to administer these funds. Although the emphasis of this act was on illegal drug usage in colleges and universities, the recognition of prevention of this problem in higher education was beginning. Legislation affecting higher education includes the following:

The Higher Education Act Amendments of 1986 required institutions receiving federal financial student aid to certify that they had drug prevention programs accessible to college administrators, employees, and students.

The Drug-Free Workplace Act of 1988 applied to all institutions that received federal grants and contracts. It required colleges and universities to achieve a drug-free workplace.

The Drug-Free Schools and Communities Act Amendments of 1989 required institutions of higher education to certify to the United States Department of Education by October 1, 1990, that they had adopted and implemented policies and programs to prevent the illicit use of drugs and the abuse of alcohol by students, faculty, and staff.

As these federal regulations were enacted by Congress, colleges and universities were required to develop policies and procedures to address the use of alcohol and other drugs. These legislative acts were being designed to support change in the campus environment. Presidents and deans of students looked for resources to develop policies, procedures, and program models. In

1987, the Secretary of Education, responding to the needs of higher education for assistance in understanding and implementing congressional mandates, brought together a group of higher education administrators under the direction of the Department of Education, Office of Educational Research and Improvement. This group developed a network to provide support for institutions that were attempting to eliminate substance abuse on their campuses. They developed a set of standards that have become known as *The Network Standards.* The Network of Colleges and Universities Committed to the Elimination of Drug and Alcohol Abuse was established by the Department of Education to provide a forum and mechanism for higher education institutions to identify and disseminate research. The standards were organized within the four areas of policy, education, enforcement, and assessment (Standards of the Network, 1988). The Network sought the participation of colleges and universities that had made a solid commitment to accomplish the following goals:

> Establish and enforce clear policies that promote an educational environment free from the abuse of alcohol and use of other drugs.
>
> Educate members of the campus community for the purpose of preventing alcohol abuse and other drug use, as well as educate them about the use of legal drugs in ways that are not harmful to themselves or to others.
>
> Create an environment that promotes and reinforces healthy, responsible living; respect for community and campus standards and regulations; the individual's responsibility within the community; and the intellectual, social, emotional, spiritual or ethical, and physical well-being of its community members.
>
> Provide for a reasonable level of care for alcohol abusers and other drug users through counseling, treatment, and referral. [Standards of the Network, 1988, p. 2]

As of 1993, 1,500 colleges and universities subscribed to these standards and had joined the network (Network of Colleges and Universities Committed to the Elimination of Drug and Alcohol Abuse, 1993). Linking the Department of Education, institutions of higher education, and national associations, the network provides leadership in assisting colleges and universities in the environmental change process.

Another resource that addresses policy issues and includes a checklist for accurate reference for policy development is *A Guide for College Presidents and Governing Boards* (Upcraft and Welty, 1990). Policies must also reflect the size, type, and culture of the institution. An appropriate policy for a large research institution would probably be inappropriate for a small private college. Knowledge of policies at similar types of colleges provides valuable information. Providing leadership and information that guides a president and the institution to develop effective policies is the appropriate role for the prevention director. Policy development should involve a committee with broad-based campus representation and with expert legal advice available as needed. Policy should be clear, simple, and consistent with federal, state, and local laws. Procedures must be developed that clearly define how the institution enforces the policy. Campuswide discussion of policy by faculty associations and other interested groups is a vital part of the process.

Finally, the policy should be approved by the governing board of the institution and disseminated to all administrators, faculty, staff, and students. Policy should be reviewed annually and revised as needed. Deans and directors who keep their president informed on policy issues and who keep their policies up-to-date influence their presidents by their knowledge and leadership.

Resource Development. A major role of all presidents is that of resource developer. State and national funding for higher education has decreased in many states in recent years. Resource development has become more important with shrinking dollars. Furthermore, since 1989, all colleges seeking federal funds are required to sign assurances of compliance with the Drug-Free Workplace Act. Therefore, prevention programs are critically important to any president interested in competing for federal dollars and in surviving federal audits. Programs either contribute to an institution's resources or drain its resources. Prevention programs that are structured to contribute to an institution's resources expand their programs and areas of influence throughout the institution.

Many colleges and universities began their institutionwide prevention programs with funds from FIPSE. These grants, while helping to initiate programs, also required institutions to commit to continue these efforts after the grant ended. Grant dollars provide an excellent source of program development money, and a creative staff will also develop strategies to secure funding from a variety of sources to continue to expand programs. Federal grants from FIPSE, Drug-Free Schools, Center for Substance Abuse Prevention (CSAP), the Department of Transportation, and the Department of Health and Human Services have been available to fund a variety of programs in colleges and universities throughout the country.

There are more needs on campuses than there are available dollars. Strategies to secure funding include a variety of tactics. Some states have provided state grants that further support programs and enhance the prevention efforts of schools in their state. A few dollars added to tuition in the form of student activities fees for substance abuse prevention programs can be an effective method for ensuring continued funding. In a college of 25,000 students, a fee of $5 each would amount to a $125,000 budget. Private and public foundations are one of the sources for program development capital. A positive relationship with the college foundation is an excellent avenue for funding. Valencia Community College's foundation collaborated with the college's prevention staff in 1989 to sponsor a major fundraising event called Kaleidoscope to which 500 community leaders came in costume for Halloween. This event featured a spectacular auction and raised a significant amount of support for the program in terms of cash and community awareness. This money, invested and matched, provides a yearly budget for items not available through other college budgets. Foundations at other colleges have developed scholarships and program funding in memory of students who have died in alcohol and drug accidents.

Revenue-producing professional education training for mental health professionals, social workers, and addiction counselors who need continuing education hours for certification or licensure satisfies both revenues enhancement and community service goals. Courses supported by full-time equivalent (FTE) and state-supported tuition meet community training needs and pay for themselves. State and national conferences and one-day workshops are options many colleges have embraced. Some colleges are working together with local elementary and secondary counselors and teachers to provide training in substance abuse issues.

Creative, innovative staff have developed numerous models that build on their institutions' expertise while developing resources, both financial and human, that range from selling program models and videos to t-shirts and posters. These professionals know how to use the available resources from organizations such as the National Clearinghouse for Alcohol and Drug Information (NCADI) and other state and national organizations.

Prevention programs often produce cost savings: legal fees, residence hall repairs, the academic loss of students who withdraw, increased security costs, and the increased burden on student health services are all costs of drug abuse on campus. Documenting these savings to the higher education CEO may turn your program into a business investment. When educational goals are met and lives are made more productive, there are savings to the institution and society. By linking national, state, and community resources of money, people, and commitment of time and talent, these college leaders are keeping the attention and commitment of their presidents and are making a difference in their college environments.

Good Press. The president is the spokesperson of the institution. Deans and directors can be of great help to the president in carrying out this role. No president can avoid questions from the community and the media about drug and alcohol issues. By providing briefing papers that contain up-to-date information that can be used to prepare speeches or in answering questions, deans and directors can keep their president informed and make it easy for him or her to be viewed as a community, state, or even national leader in addressing these problems. Deans and directors need to provide the kind of support that will make their president comfortable and confident in addressing the issues and will keep prevention information on the president's desk. Presidents need to know what the problems are on their campuses. Chapter Two, *Facts and Myths,* discusses the Core instrument that was developed to be statistically reliable and valid to assess the nature, scope, and consequences of student drug use. Presidents need to know how their institution compares to other colleges of similar kind and size in similar communities. Often, assessment information is reviewed and hidden from presidents, the student body, and the community for fear of negative public relations. Assessment measures such as the Core instrument are used to understand the campus environment. This information provides the basis for program development.

To avoid bad press, colleges often miss opportunities for good press. Survey information tied to prevention strategies provides an opportunity for positive publicity. Articles should be written in numerous school publications including alumni and foundation reports. The local newspaper will often write about innovative new programs and provide coverage about national drug and alcohol abuse weeks. Working closely with the college public relations person and the local media results in positive public relations. Prevention programs are excellent opportunities for positive press. Preventing problems also prevents bad press. Many colleges and universities face alcohol and drug tragedies that result in personal loss and negative publicity. When a crisis occurs, a well-informed president with up-to-date campus information will deal appropriately with the situation.

Strengthening the Role of the President in the Local Community. Developing good press positions the president in a community leadership role. There is not a community in America that has not been affected by drug and alcohol issues. Prevention programs offer a president the opportunity to lead the campus and community to find solutions. A Report of the Commission on the Future of Community Colleges defines community "not only as a region to be served, but also as a climate to be created" (American Association of Community and Junior Colleges, 1988, p. 7). Communities must take action to develop a healthier climate without the destructive consequences of drug and alcohol abuse. Deans and directors of prevention programs have the opportunity to encourage their presidents to participate in an active manner in community prevention. Chambers of commerce, economic development commissions, and other community groups are concerned about the consequences of substance abuse. Presidents can be educational leaders in their community by providing concerned community groups with up-to-date research and by helping these groups become proactive. Many colleges are involved in partnerships that not only provide a meeting place on campus, but assist community leaders in developing strategic action plans. Prevention staff, by working through the chain of command, can influence their president to serve on key community task forces and attend important community meetings. At Valencia Community College, the prevention staff encouraged Paul Gianini to participate on a Blue Ribbon Commission to address local drug abuse issues. The staff provided the president with background information that allowed him to assume a strong leadership role.

Community colleges were founded to be closely connected to the needs of their communities. Many four-year universities also see their educational role within local communities and define their mission to include service by establishing partnerships with the broader community. Through their leadership, presidents can become part of the solution.

College involvement in national prevention weeks such as Red Ribbon lets the community know that the college supports community prevention efforts. In an article in *Educational Record* (1989) titled "Alcohol and the Community Rethinking Privilege," David Burns states, "It seems to be our fate in this consumer culture of abundance to believe that we should blame problems on a product and then look for some other product to fix the problems. We can't shake our belief that there must be the perfect video tape, or pamphlet, or peer program, or catchy phrase, or distracting activity that will provide relief" (pp. 56–57). Burns reminds us that there is no quick fix for drug and alcohol problems. There is no product on the market that offers a miracle cure. Simply buying a consultant's time, holding a workshop, or purchasing a new videotape series will not do the job. Rather than looking for a quick and easy answer, he urges us to change the way we work together on a daily basis so that we forge stronger connections with other people—connections that build community. By focusing on improving the quality of relationships with others in our communities, we can create a climate of prevention on our campuses.

Presidents become hooked on prevention when they see the positive impact prevention programs have on their campuses and in their communities. Deans and directors who understand the role of the president can hook their presidents on prevention. Presidents can then empower the institution to fulfill its societal mission of intellectual and social learning. Institutions that incorporate prevention into their vision and culture will become the vital learning organizations of the next century.

References

American Association of Community and Junior Colleges. *Building Communities, A Vision for a New Century.* A Report of the Commission on the Future of Community Colleges. Washington, D.C.: American Association of Community and Junior Colleges, 1988.

The Drug Abuse Report. Washington, D.C.: November 1986.

Bucknam, R. B. "The Other Side of the Coin." *Journal of American College Health,* May 1994, 42, 305–307.

Burns, D. "Alcohol and the Community, Rethinking Privilege." *Educational Record,* 1989, pp. 56–57.

The Carnegie Foundation for the Advancement of Teaching. *Campus Life: In Search of Community.* Lawrenceville, N.J.: Princeton University Press, 1990, pp. 7–8, 38.

Eigen, L. D. *Alcohol Practices, Policies, and Potentials of American Colleges and Universities,* an OSAP White Paper. Rockville, Md.: National Clearinghouse for Alcohol and Drug Information, 1991, p. 1.

Lofquist, W. A. *Discovering the Meaning of Prevention.* Tucson: AYD Publications, 1989, p. 13.

Mills-Novoa, B. *Striving for Success: A Self-Assessment Guide for Strengthening Drug Prevention Programs in Higher Education.* Flagstaff: Northern Arizona University, 1992.

Presley, C. A., Meilman, P. W., and Lyerla, M. S. *Alcohol and Drugs on American College Campuses.* Volume 1: *1989–1991.* Carbondale: The Core Institute, Southern Illinois University, January 1993.

Network of Colleges and Universities Committed to the Elimination of Drug and Alcohol Abuse. *Network Directory.* Washington, D.C.: U.S. Department of Education, Office of Educational Research and Improvement, 1993.

Senge, P. M. *The Fifth Discipline.* New York: Doubleday, 1990, p. 181.

Standards of the Network of Colleges and Universities Committed to the Elimination of Drug and Alcohol Abuse. Washington, D. C.: Office of Educational Research and Improvement, 1988. (ED 292431)

Sturnick, J. A. *The Presidential Role in Alcohol and Substance Abuse Education.* Higher Education and National Affairs. Washington, D.C.: American Council on Education, July 12, 1993, p. 5.

Upcraft, M. L., and Welty, J. D. *A Guide for College Presidents and Governing Boards: Strategies for Eliminating Alcohol and Other Drug Abuse on Campuses.* Washington, D.C.: U.S. Department of Educational Research and Improvement, 1990.

Welty, J. D. *Alcohol and Other Drugs, The Changing Cultural Context.* Speech given at the Network Conference on Alcohol Abuse on College and University Campuses. Washington, D.C., November 1989.

PAUL C. GIANINI, JR., *is president of Valencia Community College and a national speaker on alcohol and drug abuse prevention in higher education.*

RUTH L. NICHOLSON *is assistant vice president of educational and economic development services at Valencia Community College and works as a consultant in developing and implementing prevention programs in higher education.*

The creation of healthy campus cultures requires reexamination
of the values, artifacts, symbols, and rituals held by student
subcultures and supported directly or indirectly by institutions
of higher education.

Students as Change Agents in Preventing Drug Abuse

D. Diane Edwards, Patricia L. Leonard

Student affairs professionals have long been committed to providing substance abuse education, and results indicate that they have been very effective in several areas. Although some may argue that efforts in alcohol education have not reduced drinking levels, the overall impact has been positive. As Dalton (1989) stated, colleges now have dry rush on campus, students routinely serve nonalcoholic beverages at social functions, staff are more sensitive about alcohol advertising and have fewer problems managing large student parties, and there is greater concern among students about safety, especially in regard to drunk driving. These changes have not occurred overnight. They have taken time and, more importantly, cooperation and collaboration among individuals, departments, divisions, and colleges to support and reinforce the need for change.

Institutions of higher education continue to struggle to change their campus environments with regard to the use of alcohol and other drugs. This task does not merely involve changing behaviors; rather, it is a matter of changing norms and attitudes. The difficulty lies in the fact that norms are not simply individual or even collective. They are an integral part of, and arise from, the cultures and communities that surround and envelop our college campuses. In this chapter, the authors will explore a different way of viewing and eventually acting upon the cultures of the collegiate environment in order to more effectively address alcohol and other drug abuse among college students.

Culture of the Institution

Part and parcel of every college or university campus is its culture, uniquely different from that of every other campus. Here, culture is defined as "persistent patterns of norms, values, practices, beliefs, and assumptions that shape the behavior of individuals and groups . . . and that provide a frame of reference within which to interpret the meaning of events and actions on and off campus" (Kuh and Whitt, 1988, p. iv). It is culture that gives events, symbols, and behaviors their meaning. This meaning or context is unique to each campus and cannot be generalized to other settings, even to other colleges or universities.

The meaning or significance of particular campus events or customs can be understood only through observing the artifacts of the institution. "Artifacts are what we can 'see' about the cultures within an institution and what we are most likely to attend to and identify when we talk about those cultures. They include history, traditions, stories, heroes and heroines, norms, symbols and interaction patterns" (Kuh, Schuh, Whitt, and Associates, 1991, p. 71). Although there may be similarities between the artifacts of several campuses, the particular "look" and practice of them can vary widely.

College Student Subcultures

Within each institution's dominant culture can be found numerous subcultures, each with a distinct membership, identity, values, behaviors, and rituals. These subcultures are essentially the peer groups described by Astin (1993, p. 400) as "a collection of individuals with whom the individual identifies and affiliates and from whom the individual seeks acceptance or approval."

College student subcultures assume a variety of appearances and often vary considerably in values, rituals, behaviors, and other distinguishing characteristics, both within and among institutions. Although at times particular subcultures have seemed to dominate our attention and are often used by the media to typify "all" college students, there has always been and will continue to be a wide range of student subcultures present on any campus (Horowitz, 1987). A clear example of this myopic view is the annual media focus on college students spending spring break on Florida beaches. Although only a small fraction of all students actually do this, the media often chooses this minority as a focus of their news coverage.

Examples of common campus student subcultures or peer groups are fraternities, sororities, cultural and minority groups, and sometimes even residents of particular buildings or floors (Dean, 1982). Other groups include women's groups, student government officers, commuting students, or nontraditional students (Roberts, 1981). Still others might include orientation leaders, intercollegiate athletes, staff members of peer educator programs, residence staff, members of close-knit clubs, and students in highly structured and time-intensive academic majors such as nursing, dance, and voice. With such diversity of subcultures present on campus, we must learn to accurately identify those on our own campuses and seek to understand what makes them tick, what they value, who their leaders are, and how they lead. From this point, we can begin to formulate ways of directly involving them in prevention work. Resident assistants, for example, must often act as disciplinarians as they enforce campus and residence policies. Some individuals are able to carry out these enforcement responsibilities equitably while maintaining excellent relations with their residents. Such students demonstrate unique and valuable leadership qualities and may be acting to change norms rather than merely behaviors. These characteristics may prove to be valuable in a subculture approach to prevention.

In his definition of peer group, Astin (1993) uses the term *acceptance* to point out two processes of group membership. First, he uses it to refer to the group's acknowledgement that the individual meets the minimum requirements for inclusion. Second, it addresses the "extent to which the individual's beliefs, conduct, and accomplishments conform to the norms and expectations of others in the group" (p. 401). Membership then is a two-way process. Students both seek membership and are selected for invitation. Dean (1982, p. 83) addresses yet another important aspect of group membership—the strength of the bond. He contends that a peer group will be "more unified and distinct the more the members believe they have values and activities in common, and a camaraderie develops."

Dean also recognizes that through the subculture selection process, potential members are accepted or rejected, creating both insiders and outsiders. This produces an environment in which "membership becomes valued and restricted" (p. 83). A clear illustration of this is the Greek system's rush and pledging process. As a result of these processes, subculture members will demonstrate a strong and shared identity through conformity to the values, norms, and expectations of the group and clear boundaries will usually exist between members and nonmembers, insiders and outsiders. Using this information, one might conclude that on a particular campus, the intramural rugby team represents a subculture, but skateboarders do not. Although members of the skateboarders' group may share similarities in dress and sport, they appear to have no clear, formal, and singular group identity. These defining characteristics clearly illustrate the power of student subcultures. As Austin points out, "the student's peer group is the single most potent source of influence on growth and development during the undergraduate years" (Astin, 1993, p. 398).

Quest to Belong

One of the most important functions of student subcultures is their role in providing members with the tools they need to negotiate the collegiate maze. Subcultures become a means of surviving or succeeding in the many arenas of campus life. As traditional-age students arrive at college, they leave behind many of the shaping influences of their communities, families, and hometown friends. Throughout their childhood and high school years, students have enjoyed the security and stability of a familiar system of rules, norms, values, and expectations learned within their communities, family, and circles of friends. However, upon graduation from high school, those old systems become less relevant and their pull less strong. The influence of home community, family, and friends weakens, leaving students with little help to negotiate challenges within their new environment. They move from being insiders within their high school subculture to outsiders on the college campus. They are, in a very real sense, in social limbo.

During this difficult transition, students search for new sources of security and stability. They look for a place to belong, for a new group of peers with whom to identify. It is common for students to initially experiment with a number of groups, eventually selecting and being selected by one or more groups with which they affiliate. In seeking and accomplishing membership in a new peer group, students often undergo changes in order to more closely conform to that group. Astin (1993, p. 398) described this accommodation by noting that "students' values, beliefs, and aspirations tend to change in the direction of the dominant values, beliefs, and aspirations of the peer group." These changes may be made before acceptance as a means of gaining membership or following admission as a way of solidifying and strengthening the bond with the new peer group.

The high level of discomfort experienced by students making the transition from high school to college and the speed with which they seek acceptance upon entering college points to the strong stabilizing effect of membership. Membership, though gained at the expense of some personal autonomy, nonetheless helps them to regain a much-needed sense of security, belonging, identity, and control. It provides the means to survive and succeed within a new environment. There is little wonder that student affairs professionals encounter resistance when trying to change a value, behavior, or symbol treasured within a student subculture, such as heavy drinking. By doing so, we are tampering with their very sense of identity. Yet this is precisely the target of many campus alcohol and other drug abuse prevention programs.

Prevention Practice: Past and Present

Alcohol and other drug abuse prevention services are relative newcomers to college campuses, with most programs being developed during the mid- to late 1980s.

Common goals of early programs included informing students of the negative effects of alcohol and other drugs and responding to actual incidents of drug abuse (by conducting floor meetings or educational programs following a weekend of alcohol-inspired vandalism, for example).

Throughout the 1980s, prevention program goals shifted toward an emphasis on educating students about responsible decision-making and the dangers of certain high-risk behaviors such as driving while impaired. On many campuses, the 1980s brought an interest in incorporating peer counselors and then peer educators into alcohol and other drug prevention programs. Research has shown that peer teaching as an educational tool positively influences learning (Pascarella and Terenzini, 1991). This positive effect extends not only to the peer teacher's student, but also to the peer teacher. Benware and Deci's 1984 study documented a "significantly higher conceptual learning of the material" (Pascarella and Terenzini, 1991, p. 99) by those who were preparing to teach it compared to those who were studying to be tested. Dean (1982) advocated the use of community developers (peer educators) specifically in alcohol and other drug abuse prevention programs. His concept was to create programs designed to deal with alcohol problems in student subgroups. He based his design on the belief that insiders within a subgroup or subculture have access to privileged information about group members and thus are better equipped to identify problems or issues within that subgroup.

By the end of the 1980s, peer education models of prevention were widely used on college campuses. Using this model, the focus turned to information dissemination. Improvisational skits were often incorporated to assist students in relating factual information about drugs and their abuse to real-life experiences, a task that too many college students are not developmentally prepared to accomplish. These approaches are still widely used today, although instructional methods have been expanded to include prevention efforts across the curriculum.

A final piece of the prevention picture has been the level of priority these services have been given on individual campuses. As indicated in Chapter Three, *Hooking Your President on Prevention*, the active endorsement of the college or university president is important to the prominence and success of the program. The organization of prevention services also affects the program's effectiveness. On some campuses, alcohol and other drug abuse prevention services are the sole responsibility of one office. However, more often than not, the primary responsibility for alcohol and other drug prevention is placed within an office as only one of several functions. This effectively limits the quantity, quality, and variety of prevention services. As a result of centralization, few other campus offices assume responsibility for providing prevention services. If Penny Norton, project director of Facing Alcohol Concerns Through Education (FACE) is correct in her contention that prevention professionals must "hit, hit, hit" students with clear prevention messages, then the usual output of many centralized service providers may not be sufficient in quantity or consistency to be effective. In order to counter the strong influence of the peer subculture, prevention messages must be pervasive and absolutely consistent throughout the campus.

In theory, the centralization of services may have been desirable during the early years of campus prevention work. However, shrinking budgets of the 1990s may soon make that approach impractical as prevention professionals are forced to take on additional responsibilities. Ever-tightening budgets for student services may soon force prevention professionals to rethink the way they do their jobs, moving away from acting on students one-to-one toward acting from within subcultures themselves. With many college prevention programs now completing their building years and entering a new phase of service development and enhancement, the time may now be right for a shift in prevention theory, goals, and methods.

Prospects for Change

Clearly, rituals and other cultural artifacts have tremendous potential for exerting a positive influence on student behavior and the campus environment. In the case of alcohol and other drug use, the dominant college student subculture on campuses often approves and encourages use in ways that differ markedly from those deemed appropriate by prevention professionals. It is in this arena that the institutional culture and the student subcultures often clash. Over the past ten years of high-intensity campus prevention programming, that clash has left university administrators and prevention professionals picking themselves up off the ground and shaking their heads, amazed that student resistance to any change can be so intense.

However, student affairs professionals must remember two points. First, behavioral change occurs slowly, usually over months or years. Second, the campus environment itself places students at high risk for the abuse of alcohol and other drugs. Both are significant factors to consider in developing and implementing prevention programs. However, the subcultures themselves, by their very nature, may give prevention professionals opportunities for introducing change. According to G. Morgan, cultures are "constantly evolving, incorporating changes in the values, beliefs and attitudes of the external environment as well as those of institutional members" (Kuh, Schuh, Whitt, and Associates, 1991, p. 71). If this is true, then significant and lasting change in alcohol and other drug use should be a realistic goal. The evolving nature of culture may present a much-needed window of opportunity for change in alcohol and other drug use behaviors.

Constructing a New Perspective

It is doubtful that any effort for change imposed by authority figures from outside the peer subculture will have any significant impact. Change must begin where students find themselves validated, where they gain their sense of worth and their framework for assessing behaviors. That place is their peer subculture. If Dalton (1989, p. 184) is correct in his assertion that "alcohol use is at the heart of peer culture," then it is that culture as a whole that must be the focus of prevention efforts. Butler (1993) clearly pinpoints that focus on artifacts that bear significance for students, such as their rituals, rites of passage, and folklore.

Case for Prevention Through Systems Influence

Methods of alcohol and other drug abuse prevention such as those mentioned earlier provide a valuable starting point from which to rethink and redesign prevention practices. What is needed first, however, is an expanded field of influence.

There are two critical priorities for campus alcohol and other drug prevention in coming years: prevention efforts must be directed toward changing the peer subculture, its values, norms, and artifacts; and prevention professionals must develop and implement ways to improve the clarity and consistency of alcohol and other drug abuse prevention messages, multiply the number of messages, and increase the frequency with which students receive them.

Addressing these needs will require a shift in perspective, from focusing on individuals to acting from within the larger peer culture. If change can begin from within the peer subculture, then broader, more significant, and more lasting shifts in student behaviors and attitudes will likely follow.

Applying Systems Thinking in Prevention Practices

Systems thinking, or the systems approach, to alcohol and other drug prevention requires first a thorough understanding of the system or subsystem to be addressed. To begin to apply systems thinking to campus prevention practice, one must recognize that within the peer subsystem there exists a range of other subcultures or subsystems. One must also understand some of the dominant characteristics of peer cultures.

In order to apply systems thinking to prevention, we must address the priorities set forth in the previous section. We must determine the desired changes in norms, values, attitudes, and behaviors related to alcohol and other drug use; identify the members of the peer culture or subsystem who are most influential within that culture; and build upon the peer teaching model by incorporating prevention artifacts, traditions, and symbols into educational programs and activities to communicate the desired changes in tangible and relevant ways.

The definition and design of the desired learning is a critical step in bringing about change in the peer culture, but the focus here will be on developing the means of delivering that message to specific subcultures.

Cultural Artifacts and Alcohol and Other Drug Use

Despite all the positive contributions to the institution and to the lives and success of students, it is within college student subcultures that many of the most persistent and potentially harmful behaviors are promoted and actively reinforced as norms. Often-expected or sanctioned behaviors such as binge drinking can provide powerful resistance to change largely due to the strength of influence of the subcultures.

This is especially true of first-year traditional college-age students. Usually away from the watchful eye of family and friends for the first time, first-year students are likely to act in very conformist ways by bending to fit their desired peer group's definition of successful membership. A student subculture's approval and encouragement of certain behaviors are powerful reinforcing mechanisms and use a number of measures to teach and perpetuate desired actions. A common example might include morning-after stories where the previous night's behavior is the central focus of student laughter and positive reinforcement.

One means of defining, giving meaning to, and thus teaching a subculture's sanctioned behaviors is through honoring of the culture's rituals, folklore, traditions, or customs. Bronner (1990, p. 204) described clearly the role of these cultural artifacts: "students share folklore with their peers to reflect on matters of sex, courtship, fidelity, drugs, and security. . . . Through folklore, students confront their cultural status and that of others according to gender, race, religion, occupation, age, and class."

Rituals and rites of passage in particular are important tools in assisting students through the difficult transitions between adolescence and adulthood (Butler, 1993). A significant part of many of the subcultures' rituals, traditions, and folklore is the use of alcohol and other drugs. According to Burda and Vaux (1988), alcohol and other drug use plays an important role in college male bonding and in students proving their preparedness for membership in certain subcultures and as adults (Butler, 1993). Initiation rites involving coercion such as those practiced among some fraternal organizations and within some campus military programs are perhaps some of the best-known examples. Other examples common among tight-knit groups are chants, cheers, and drinking games that encourage excessive and usually rapid consumption of alcohol. A common practice among some club sports, such as rugby, is for the host team to sponsor a party where the main activity is excessive drinking. In the rugby subculture, this is considered a sacred ritual.

Campus legends and lore also help define what is perceived as acceptable and admired use of alcohol and other drugs (Bronner, 1990). Some prescribe predrinking regimens, others describe the feats of folk heroes who exemplify excessive alcohol use, and still others dictate rituals for significant milestones, such as drinking shots to celebrate a twenty-first birthday or getting drunk after a big test. Campus graffiti also communicates a variety of messages about alcohol and other drug use. One example given by Bronner (1990, p. 203) was "Reality is for people who can't handle drugs." There are endless examples of rituals students use to signify and solidify their membership in a particular student subculture. Prevention professionals and others on college campuses must gain an intimate understanding of these rituals and work toward helping students develop new and "meaningful but harmless rites of passage rituals" (Butler, 1993, p. 53).

Understanding Student Artifacts

The first step is determining the desired changes in the campus culture. This might be accomplished by adding one or two questions to the self-assessment guide provided in Chapter Seven, *Striving for Success*. A sample question might be, "What campus rituals affect students' attitudes on our campus toward alcohol and other drug use?" One example of such a ritual might be tailgating before football games. Other examples or areas to be examined are the activities of new student orientation programs, the training of resident assistants for their first floor meetings of the year, and the advertising guidelines for campus activities. Overall, what are the standards and expectations of student behavior on your campus and how and when are they communicated?

Another way to gain an understanding of campus artifacts and rituals might be through meetings with groups of students to discuss their lives and lifestyles. Possible formats for these meetings could be focus groups or town halls. This type of event should be developed and conducted by student subculture leaders. Such meetings could be implemented as part of a student's practicum experience under the supervision of a supportive faculty member.

An extension of the town hall idea is a showcase for different student groups. Representatives from a variety of student subcultures, both formal and informal, are invited to share with the campus community some of their unique characteristics. This might be conducted much like a cultural fair but with more structure to ensure that the purpose of gathering information is accomplished. The actual information-gathering could be carried out by teams of students, faculty, and administrators, each responsible for collecting information on the artifacts and symbols of the various groups. Information from either of these types of events could then be compiled into a directory of artifacts, each examined for its role in student-to-student and student-to-university bonding and its impact on student alcohol and other drug use.

Getting Inside Subcultures

What is known about student subcultures is based largely on professional observation and on our often well-aged recollection of our own college years. Our challenge is to gain a more accurate perspective by seeking an insider's access to current student subcultures. Prevention professionals have years of experience and research in reacting to negative behaviors, yet we have little or no precedent for helping students initiate proactive and positive change from within their subcultures. Without prototypes to follow, student affairs professionals will need to openly explore new approaches and try creative new ideas for affecting student subcultures.

One long-standing means for gaining entry into student subcultures is peer education. Students selected for these roles are often brought in through the traditional job recruitment, application, and selection process. These individuals in most cases self-identify and, as a result, may not always provide an accurate representation of the existing student subcultures. Although they may not be true subculture leaders, their role in prevention is valuable. These peer educators should be guided into prevention education activities most appropriate to their expertise and interests.

If the goal is to gain that insider's access to student subcultures, then prevention professionals should attempt to identify members of the peer culture with the greatest potential for influence on that culture. The identification of those key, highly influential students begins with a close look at both the peer culture and the broader campus culture. The task is to identify individual students and groups of students who, by their positioning or visibility, can initiate change from within subcultures. *Positioning* here refers to the point and timing of contact peer leaders have with critical segments of the student culture. Student orientation leaders and resident assistants, for example, are uniquely positioned to be among the first individuals new students meet. Because we know that the first six weeks of the freshman year are critical in setting the tone for student success, these leaders may present opportunities for subculture access earlier than any other formal student group.

Highly influential students vary from campus to campus and are dictated by the individual centers of power on each campus. Some may be persons in positions traditionally labeled as student leaders such as resident assistants, orientation leaders, student government officers, peer educators, fraternity and sorority officers, and members of high-profile organizations such as GAMMA (Greeks Advocating Mature Management of Alcohol) and BACCHUS (Boost Alcohol Consciousness Concerning the Health of University Students). Other students who may be very closely tied to the peer culture but may not hold traditional campus leadership positions include intramural team captains, campus union employees, staff members of student-run television and radio stations, and informal leaders in residence halls or off-campus housing complexes. Any of these individuals may be valuable allies in gaining access to student subcultures.

Building New Artifacts, Traditions, and Symbols

After identifying the desired changes and subculture leaders, the process of reshaping of subculture values, artifacts, and rituals can begin. Programs for new students that introduce them to values, norms, behaviors, and standards appropriate to membership in the academic community of their chosen institution are a logical beginning for such restructuring. These new symbols might include new-student commencement ceremonies in which students receive the "book of knowledge" for the college or university. This "book of knowledge" could include the values of the institution such as a commitment to friendliness characterized by an institution-specific greeting shared on campus. New students might be assigned academic mentors and receive transition artifacts that carry the University motto. African-American students might be introduced to culturally specific symbols such as the kinte cloth with the goal that upon graduation they will receive the cloth from a faculty mentor.

Many of the often negative practices mentioned earlier in this chapter would serve as excellent starting points for developing what Butler referred to as "meaningful but harmless rites of passage rituals" (Butler, 1993, p. 53). Resident assistants might institute a variety of hall-wide celebrations to recognize students' milestones such as reaching one's twenty-first birthday, completing a test, or gaining acceptance into selective student groups. Club sports teams such as rugby (which sometimes attempts to create an "outlaw" identity in order to gain status) could be given the same recognition and praise heaped on certain intercollegiate teams, including celebrations to mark tournament success or advancement toward state, regional, or national titles. Even graffiti could be purposely created to convey very specific and positive messages about student life. The element that each of these has in common is that they emphasize, recognize, praise, and make visible that which is good among our students. The possibilities are limitless. But first we must realize that initiating or changing institutional artifacts and communicating the institution's values, norms, and expectations are our responsibilities as educators.

Once new rites of passage have been established, the consistency of the messages they carry must be evaluated. The task of communicating cultural norms cannot be left up to traditional orientation programs that whisk students quickly in and out. Activities should be planned to occur beginning with high school graduation throughout the summer and during the entire first year to ensure both initiation and assimilation into the campus culture. Faculty members, for example, might develop rituals for their individual classes to mark the start of the academic year or the end of the semester. Student representatives of all major campus subculture constituencies could be challenged to develop appropriate symbols representing the values that have been endorsed by the institution.

Finally, it is critical that, as we shift toward a systems approach to prevention, we acknowledge the power, worth, and contribution of the individual student subcultures. Failure to generously credit these systems for the meaning and value they have for students seriously limits our ability to build new artifacts, symbols, and traditions and to initiate change within those subcultures.

The Future

The goal of this chapter has been to challenge all student affairs professionals, especially those involved with alcohol and other drug abuse prevention, to look more closely at our own campuses and student subcultures for windows of opportunity. What we have proposed requires that we stretch beyond the familiar, that we be willing to chart new territory, and that we look to a different arena in which to begin introducing change. This stretch is a risk for us and for our institutions. Chances are good that we will uncover some unpleasant truths about ourselves, both personally and institutionally, such as steps that we could have taken and did not. To make this stretch, we must be willing to learn about ourselves, our students, and our institutions, and to use what we learn to create more positive and life-enhancing campus environments. We believe that a systems approach such as the one proposed here brings with it greater prospects for positive change than campuses have previously enjoyed. The time has come for prevention work on campuses to move to the next level of development, a level that brings to our field an excitement and promise whose time has arrived.

References

Astin, A. W. *What Matters in College? Four Critical Years Revisited.* San Francisco: Jossey-Bass, 1993, pp. 398–401.

Benware, C., and Deci, E. "Quality of Learning with an Active Versus Passive Motivational Set." *American Educational Research Journal,* 1984, *21,* 755–765.

Bronner, S. J. *Piled Higher and Deeper, The Folklore of Campus Life.* Little Rock, Ark.: August House, 1990, pp. 123, 124, 192, 203, 204.

Burda, P. C., and Vaux, A. C. "Social Drinking in Support Contexts Among College Males." *Journal of Youth and Adolescence,* 1988, *17* (2), 165–171.

Butler, E. R. "Alcohol Use by College Students: A Rites of Passage Ritual." *NASPA Journal,* Fall 1993, *31,* 48–55.

Dalton, J. C. "The Influence of Peer Culture on College Student Values." *NASPA Journal,* Spring 1989, *26* (3), 180–186.

Dean, J. C. *Approaches to Alcohol Abuse Prevention.* In J. C. Dean and W. A. Bryan (eds.), *Alcohol Programming for Higher Education.* Carbondale: ACPA Media, Southern Illinois University Press, 1982, pp. 30, 82–84.

Horowitz, H. L. *Campus Life Undergraduate Cultures from the End of the Eighteenth Century to the Present.* New York: Knopf, 1987.

Kuh, G. D., Schuh, J. H., Whitt, E. J., and Associates. *Involving Colleges Successful Approaches to Fostering Student Learning and Development Outside the Classroom.* San Francisco: Jossey-Bass, 1991, pp. 71–72.

Kuh, G. D., and Whitt, E. J. *The Invisible Tapestry: Culture in American Colleges and Universities.* AAHE-ERIC/Higher Education Research Report no. 1. Washington, D.C.: American Association for Higher Education, 1988, p. iv.

Pascarella, E. T., and Terenzini, P. J. *How College Affects Students: Findings and Insights from Twenty Years of Research.* San Francisco: Jossey-Bass, 1991, p. 99.

Roberts, D. C. (ed.). *Student Leadership Programs in Higher Education.* Carbondale: ACPA Media, Southern Illinois University Press, 1981, p. 112.

D. DIANE EDWARDS *is coordinator of Alternatives! alcohol and other drug education and prevention services at the University of North Carolina at Wilmington. She also coordinates campus sexual assault education services.*

PATRICIA L. LEONARD *is the dean of students at the University of North Carolina at Wilmington.*

Prevention across the curriculum is a new application of a proven technique. This cost-effective approach to alcohol and other drug use prevention is particularly effective on commuter campuses.

Prevention Across the Curriculum

Emily C. Wadsworth, John R. Hoeppel, R. Kipp Hassell

It is the intent of this chapter to describe curriculum infusion, a prevention strategy that is particularly effective on commuter campuses. Faculty design modules for their own courses in which the prevention information fits seamlessly with the scholarly content and students actively process that information. By working with someone in academic affairs to identify courses, recruit and train faculty, and maintain faculty interest, student affairs personnel are able to build lasting bridges with academic affairs.

Curriculum infusion as a prevention strategy can be thought of as prevention across the curriculum, which will have a familiar ring to the faculty. As early as the 1970s, "writing across the curriculum" and "critical thinking across the curriculum" programs encouraged faculty to involve their students in actively processing the content of their courses. Faculty development and instructional development specialists have long been working with faculty to improve their teaching by encouraging them to use varied and interactive teaching strategies. The literature on teaching and learning abounds with articles and research demonstrating the need for both greater variety in teaching strategies and greater student involvement with the content. Jonathan Fife, in the foreword to a 1991 ASHE–ERIC Higher Education Report, points out that "[i]ncreasingly, college and university faculty are being held accountable for the effectiveness of their teaching. Research has clearly demonstrated that the more college students become involved with the education process, the more they learn. . . . The concept of active learning—that is, increasing students' involvement in the learning process—is an indispensable technique for increasing the effectiveness of teaching" (Bonwell and Eison, 1991, Foreword).

From this perspective, one of the most effective prevention strategies is to ask students to apply information about the effects of substance use to their own lives. In fact, one might conjecture that it is only when an individual becomes aware of the potential effect of substance use on his or her life that attitudes and behavior change. Bruce Joleaud suggests that "[p]roviding accurate information about alcohol and drugs so that people actively use the information as they make decisions about their lives" is one of the most powerful prevention strategies (Hoeppel and Wadsworth, 1992, p. 62). Curriculum infusion engages students in actively learning about substance use and abuse within the regular scholarly content of an existing course. Thus, curriculum infusion promotes both excellent teaching and effective prevention by requiring active engagement with the subject matter.

Curriculum infusion is a significant contribution to the array of prevention activities on campus. All students take classes. Regardless of their cultural diversity, their different needs, different goals, and different ages, they all meet in the classroom. Using the faculty and their classrooms as the stage for prevention initiatives, it is possible to reach each student in the institution, and reach them in a naturalistic setting where the prevention message can be delivered in a content-appropriate way. The curriculum infusion model for prevention programming uses this classroom connection.

Of course, prevention across the curriculum must be combined with the strategies more typically provided by student affairs programs: workshops, student activities fairs, orientation sessions, and college awareness days. "Research has repeatedly shown that out-of-class experience has a major impact on college students—emotionally, socially, morally, and physically as well as mentally" (Chickering, A., and Associates, 1981, p. 657). Thus, a combination of classroom-based and cocurricular strategies makes prevention a part of the daily lives of students just as substance abuse is often a part of their daily lives.

There are, of course, other forms of curriculum infusion. In one version, the prevention program supports a campus speakers' bureau. Instead of canceling class at times when they are unable to attend, faculty can request a prevention speaker. This model has the potential to reach many students in many different courses, but carries the disadvantage of having the prevention message seen as an add-on to the regular curriculum. Another curriculum infusion model adds prevention as a course or part of a course in substance abuse treatment majors or health and wellness majors. Here the disadvantage is that students have self-selected into the major or program, and hence the institution is likely to miss the average student.

Definitions

Prevention across the curriculum includes information about substance use and abuse in an academic course so that the prevention material fits seamlessly with the normal scholarly content of the course. The weaving of prevention material into an existing course is the essence of the curriculum infusion model. This is often accomplished through the development of course modules on prevention. A module is a replaceable course element that occupies a specific amount of class time (at least two weeks, for instance) and presents prevention-based content in a manner that employs active learning—that is, it engages students in collecting, analyzing, evaluating, and using information, rather than passively receiving it. The development of the module is informed and driven by a knowledge of prevention strategies, assessment data about the target problems on the particular campus, substance abuse information, and pedagogical techniques. Figure 5.1 depicts in a graphic way the influences that combine to form the curriculum infusion model. Much of the material that forms this chapter is an amplification of the ideas implicit in this model. A detailed guide to establishing a curriculum infusion approach to prevention efforts is available elsewhere (Hoeppel and Wadsworth, 1992).

Depending on its design, a course module can be used in several courses and may be repeatable in later offerings of the same course. What is critical is that prevention material be interwoven in the academic fabric of the course seamlessly so that its influence is indirect and doesn't interrupt the formal course objectives. In actual use, many faculty members remark that the development of active-learning prevention modules helps students learn better because they become more involved in the learning process. Many faculty with whom the authors have worked also report that their teaching changes to include more active learning strategies.

Figure 5.1. Substance Abuse Prevention: Curriculum Infusion Model

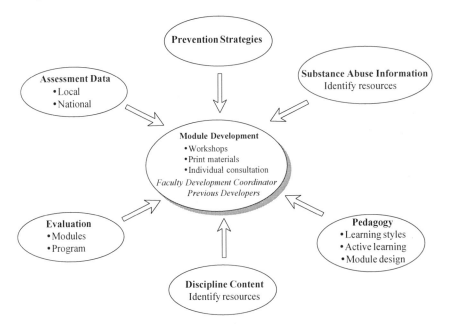

Curriculum infusion involves a partnership with the faculty, a bridge between academic and student affairs. Student affairs professionals provide expertise in prevention and support to the faculty as the faculty provide expertise in their disciplines and actually bring the prevention message to the students. Once student affairs professionals have built the bridge with faculty through curriculum infusion, faculty often participate more actively in other student affairs projects.

How does this work? As an example, students in a newswriting course prepared a four-page supplement to the school newspaper on substance use and abuse. The nominal focus of this activity was journalism and newswriting; the secondary impact on students was the content-based prevention material that had been woven into the fabric of the course.

In a general introduction to philosophy course, the students read the article "Drunk Driving" by philosopher Connie Steinbock (Steinbock, 1985). The article deals with three issues: are DUI killings murder? Can alcoholics be held responsible for their DUI actions? What are fair punishments for DUI killings/offenses? The students discuss the three issues in units on morality and ethics, freedom and determinism, morality, and social and political issues. In addition to class discussion, students do library research to gather data relating to DUIs and write a short paper addressing the issues from one of the three areas of thought. Although the philosophical perspective and reasoning process form the primary focus of this activity, the students apply critical, logical reasoning processes to a substance abuse issue. The selection of subject matter influences what students think about, learn about, and discuss with their friends in a more thoughtful, thorough manner. In the above example, students discuss, research, and think about the ethical issues related to driving under the influence of alcohol or other drugs. This is why curriculum infusion is so effective—it reaches students with prevention material in a naturalistic way, often while they are learning about something else.

Building Bridges

Because it is classroom-based, curriculum infusion demands collaboration with the faculty. In fact, curriculum infusion is about student affairs building bridges to student lives through the faculty. The curriculum infusion model is cost-effective, potentially reaching all students through existing structures in a low-cost, significant way. It is cost-efficient because the efforts tend to be one-time investments that produce products and expertise used again and again. A course-based delivery strategy for prevention programming also targets a guaranteed audience, in contrast to student affairs' more common experience of working hard to attract the already over-committed and over-stressed student. Working closely with the faculty can build positive benefits that carry over into support and enhanced understanding for other student affairs initiatives.

Students come and go; it is the faculty who form the most stable populations on our campuses. Faculty tend to remain at an institution for long periods of time, once tenured, often for the rest of their careers. Hence, bridges built between student affairs and faculty members tend to be long-lived. Committed faculty members use curriculum infusion over many years and in many of their classes.

Prevention across the curriculum is particularly effective in community colleges and urban universities where students commute. The model can, however, be used in other institutional settings, even the most prestigious research universities. For example, Harvard, Stanford, Northwestern, the University of Wisconsin System, the University of California at Berkeley, and many others all have some version of a teaching and learning center designed to work with faculty to improve their teaching.

Examples

To explain how curriculum infusion works, some hypothetical scenarios are useful. Each of these scenarios contains elements from actual practice.

Example 1. Dr. Gray teaches an introductory biology course and anatomy and physiology for allied health professionals at a community college. He is a member of the curriculum council and an officer of the faculty association. Several years ago, the dean of student affairs persuaded Dr. Gray to set aside twenty minutes at the end of the class period during the first week of class for the director of health services to administer the college's substance abuse prevention needs assessment to the students in his class. Using the results of the survey, the director of health services was able to interest Dr. Gray in developing a prevention module for his anatomy and physiology course. The module was so successful that Dr. Gray now also uses the college speakers' forum to invite a speaker to his biology classes to discuss fetal alcohol syndrome during Alcohol Awareness Week. Dr. Gray is now also a member of the Committee for Substance Abuse Prevention and has persuaded other faculty members to develop modules and to participate in collegiate prevention weeks.

Additionally, almost every time the needs assessment is administered in Dr. Gray's classes, at least one student follows the administrator of the survey back to her office to inquire about help for a substance abuse–related problem. Many of Dr. Gray's students are adults who are planning additions to their families. After the lecture on fetal alcohol syndrome, students ask for further information for themselves or their significant others. In his anatomy and physiology class, Dr. Gray asks students to keep diaries for two weeks of everything they eat and drink. At the end of the two weeks, they choose one thing that they eat or drink regularly and eliminate it from their diet. Through this exercise, they learn how their patients may respond when they prescribe or work with patients whose physicians have prescribed a major change in their diets. Students who choose to eliminate alcohol, caffeine, or nicotine also experience their own struggle with eliminating a chemical substance from their lives.

Example 2. Sally Smith is a typical first-year student at a residential college. In her introductory psychology course, she gathers information about why and how people use substances at various stages in the life cycle. In her introductory speech communication course, she reads and analyzes a case study about a student who abuses alcohol on campus and comes before the student disciplinary board for a hearing. In the unit on statistics in her mathematics course, she analyzes the data from the student needs assessment as one of her assignments. The Guerrilla Theater Prevention Troupe presents skits to her sorority on acquaintance rape, alcohol use, and AIDS. In her second semester, Sally becomes interested in student activities and participates in a student activities leadership training workshop where she learns leadership and communication skills.

Example 3. Sam Smith, Sally's brother, is in his junior year majoring in business. In his introductory management class, he learns how, as a manager, to identify and work with employees who are substance abusers. In his human relations course, he learns the role substance abusers can play in creating dissension among employees. As a class assignment, he designs an employee assistance program that includes help for substance abusers. In his finance course, he learns the cost to the firm of employee substance abuse.

In a composition class, the instructor used substance abuse as the subject matter of sample essays for each of the writing assignments. While the students were learning the principles of good writing, they were also learning about substance abuse. In an acting course, students developed short skits involving substance use and its ramifications, such as acquaintance rape. They then produced the skits for various groups on and off campus. Both the student actors and the members of the audience learned more about substance abuse from the point of view of the students themselves, as it is the student actors who created the skits.

In an introductory mass communications course, the instructor required students to keep a log of television beer and wine ads. The log asked students to identify the program, the characteristics of the audience, and the message of the ads. Students discovered that the ads suggested that in order to have a good party and to be "with it," one must drink wine or beer. Many students in the course were angry because they felt as if they were being manipulated by the liquor companies and took another look at their own use of alcohol. Their reactions clearly illustrate the results of collecting, analyzing, evaluating, and using the prevention information infused into this course.

As is evident in these examples, curriculum infusion includes information about substance use and abuse in courses in such a way that the information fits seamlessly with the academic content of the courses and in such a way that the students collect, analyze, evaluate, and use the information. Other examples hint at the variety of ways in which curriculum infusion can be implemented in courses across the institution.

The key to implementing an effective curriculum infusion plan is bridging the gap between academic and student affairs. Quite often, professionals in the worlds of academic and student affairs operate in different arenas with different assumptions. As student affairs professionals develop their curriculum infusion plan, strong personal bridges are often established between the key players. This added benefit of the curriculum infusion model is that once a strong bridge to the faculty has been built, it can be used to bring faculty closer to a student development perspective in their teaching and relationships with students.

Key Implementation Steps

Choosing a project coordinator. It is imperative to identify a faculty development coordinator who has the ability to be a change agent and ensure completion of the project. This person should be someone who is already respected by the faculty for his or her good teaching or knowledge of good teaching. Many colleges have faculty development offices or committees that can recommend someone. That person will be persuaded to join the prevention effort because of an abiding interest in good teaching and the welfare of students. The faculty development coordinator will need to be compensated in a fashion appropriate to his or her position in the institution. However, the faculty development specialists may well take the project on as part of their jobs. Teaching faculty can be compensated with release time, summer employment, overload pay, or whatever is valued in the particular institution.

Scholarly information about the extent of substance use among college students based on the Johnston survey (Johnston, O'Malley, and Bachman, 1991) or the actual needs assessment data from the specific institution is useful in persuading someone to take on the task of developing the curriculum infusion project. On commuter campuses, data about the percentage of students who are living in families with substance abuse problems add to the strength of the argument. Finally, monetary or time rewards to faculty and funds for workshops on teaching as well as honorific recognition are critical to demonstrating institutional commitment to the program.

It is not necessary for the faculty development coordinator to have any expertise in substance abuse prevention except to know that, as with all teaching, the most effective method of prevention is for the audience to interact actively with the information (Bonwell and Eison, 1991; Johnson, Johnson, and Smith, 1991; Sivinicki, 1990). A good faculty development coordinator will already know how to work with the faculty and how to persuade them to participate in the project. They will need to know the elements that faculty need to know in order to design and implement a module.

Selecting target courses. The faculty development coordinator's first consideration will be selecting courses and faculty to target for modules. To maximize the impact of available resources, the project will ideally reach the greatest number of students possible in as many different cohorts of students possible.

This means that the faculty development coordinator will want to analyze and "unbundle" the student body to determine when they enter and when they leave. Some schools have large cohorts of first- and second-year students who transfer to other schools for their majors. In that case, the project should target general education courses. In community colleges, many students enroll in occupational or applied degree programs in which very few general education courses are required for graduation. In this case, the best choice will be the general education course and required courses or other high-traffic sections taken by those students. Finally, at some institutions, students transfer in during their junior year to complete a major. In this case, the program will reach the largest number of students by targeting the required courses in the most popular major.

Recruiting faculty. Having developed a list of target courses, the faculty development coordinator will want to match these courses with a list of the most respected faculty in the institution. Those faculty need to be respected by the students for their teaching and by the faculty for their scholarly knowledge and participation in the faculty governance of the institution. In other words, the faculty development coordinator is looking for faculty opinion leaders. The target faculty's good teaching will ensure the success of the modules. The target faculty's position as opinion leaders will create legitimacy for the program and make recruiting subsequent faculty easier.

Before approaching the faculty, the faculty development coordinator should work out the incentives and expectations for faculty participation. The incentives can include recognition, release time, money, a student assistant, or goods (travel funds, books, films). The expectations usually include attending a series of workshops and designing, writing up, implementing, and evaluating the module.

The incentives must be valued by the faculty at that institution. Often the most valuable form of recognition for faculty is something that will count toward retention, promotion, or tenure. In this case, it is important to work with the chief academic officer, the deans, and department chairs to get a commitment that the work on the module can be included on the faculty member's *curriculum vitae,* preferably in the research category. Other forms of recognition include honorific lunches, mention in newsletters, and honorific memos from the chief academic officer.

A survey of faculty or deans and department chairs can identify faculty who already have expertise in substance use and abuse programs. These faculty are often useful as resource people for other faculty. They tend, however, to be knowledgeable about intervention and treatment rather than prevention. They also may not teach the kinds of general education courses that reach many students.

Building capacity of the faculty to design modules. Before approaching the target faculty, the faculty development coordinator will want to be quite specific about what the faculty will need to know in order to design and implement a module and how this information will be presented to the faculty. The most common methods of presentation are printed materials and workshops. Faculty will need general information about substance use in the United States, current information about substance use nationally and among the student body, prevention strategies, active teaching and learning strategies, and module evaluations.

A series of four two-hour workshops with accompanying print materials works well (Hoeppel and Wadsworth, 1992). While providing necessary content information to the faculty, these capacity-building workshops can also serve as models of how substance use and abuse issues can be explored and discussed in a learning context.

In the first workshop, a knowledgeable faculty member can present a brief history of substance use in the United States, leading to a presentation of the results of the on-campus needs assessment. The presenter must be prepared to defend the survey design, the meaning assigned to the items, and the statistical analysis. It is the nature of many in the faculty to question; presentations on this issue will be no exception. For example, faculty are likely to ask why five drinks at a sitting is considered binge drinking: who decided five and not three or six drinks at a sitting represents binge drinking, and what are the negative effects of binge drinking? They will want to know who took the survey and under what circumstances. They will question the self-report nature of the survey. Faculty may also question the best response to the problems identified by the survey. For example, they may suggest that students binge drink because there is nothing else to do and that the appropriate response here is to provide more interesting activities for student participation rather than developing modules. The individual presenting this first faculty development workshop must be prepared to engage the faculty in lively discussion that can serve as an example of good teaching. Responding to these concerns of the faculty is essential to enlisting their collaboration and enthusiasm, in much the same way that responding to students' concerns is critical to engaging them in the learning process.

The predominant teaching technique in most colleges and universities is the lecture. For both prevention and good teaching purposes faculty need to vary their teaching techniques to include active learning experiences for the students. One good way to persuade faculty to include variety in their teaching methods is to present a workshop on learning styles; the second session in this faculty development series is an ideal place to explore this topic. Even the best teachers tend to teach the way they learn most comfortably. A learning styles workshop reminds the faculty that there are people who learn more comfortably in other modes and provides an opportunity for the faculty to begin developing their own module. David Kolb's learning styles inventory (Chickering and Associates, 1981) is particularly useful for this kind of workshop. Faculty can take the inventory and then divide into groups of faculty with either similar or different learning styles. These groups of faculty would develop a series of student prevention assignments that take students around the learning cycle.

By the time module developers reach the third workshop, they should have some idea of how they will approach prevention in their course. This is the workshop in which the faculty development coordinator should ask the faculty to share their ideas and to get feedback from other faculty in the group. This is also the time to talk about nitty-gritty issues such as writing up and evaluating the module. The module write-up should ask faculty to identify the learning goals, the prevention rationale, the content, the learning activities used to teach the content, and the evaluation method. The group itself may want to identify some common questions to ask students about their response to the module in terms of behavior and attitude change and strengths and weaknesses of the module.

In addition to asking students to evaluate each module, the faculty development coordinator will want to get feedback from the faculty themselves. The following are some possible questions for a module developer's survey:

Summarize the positive aspects of your project.
Summarize the negative aspects of your project.
Will you use your curriculum infusion model in the same course in the future? Why or why not?
What changes would you make in your project before using the material again?
Will you use your module in other courses that you teach? Which ones?
What were the most and least beneficial aspects of the training you received about curriculum infusion?
Summarize your impressions of how the students reacted to your project.

The final workshop in the series might take the form of an honorific lunch with a featured speaker and the opportunity for faculty to share their successes with each other. This is also a good time to include faculty who have developed modules in previous years or who are on a substance abuse prevention advisory committee.

The faculty development coordinator should also provide print materials for the module developers. The Network for the Dissemination of Curriculum Infusion produces a newsletter, *Network News* (for more information, contact the Network for the Dissemination of Curriculum Infusion at Northeastern Illinois University in Chicago at 312–794–6697). Each issue of the newsletter contains a reproducible essay on teaching that is directed to the faculty. It can also be distributed to former module developers to keep them interested or to the entire faculty to generate interest.

An annotated bibliography of materials in the institution's library and distribution by the faculty development coordinator of some of the best articles on prevention and teaching will keep the interest of faculty. Examples of prevention modules and evaluation comments should be made available to current developers. Faculty interest can also be maintained by annually distributing the needs assessment survey results to all former module developers as well as surveying them to discover how they are currently using the materials they developed.

Long-term follow through. Students come and go, but many of the faculty remain at the institution for much of their working lives. Therefore, the project coordinator will want to keep in touch with module developers. Many faculty participate in prevention in other ways such as including prevention class sessions during prevention awareness weeks, using part or all of their module in more than one course, serving on a prevention advisory committee, and administering the needs assessment in their courses. Some faculty may ask that the needs assessment be administered at the beginning of a class period with the remainder of the time devoted to a discussion of student response to the survey bolstered by the results of the previous year. In addition to sharing print materials with former module developers, faculty development coordinators will want to include them in some of the activities for current module developers. If funds are available to provide a new teaching and learning workshop, the faculty development coordinator will want to invite past as well as current module developers. Faculty can share especially successful modules with current developers or talk about the process they used to develop their own module. All of these things keep module developers interested and encourage them to use and to expand their original module.

References

Bonwell, C., and Eison, J. *Active Learning: Creating Excitement in the Classroom.* ASHE–ERIC Higher Education Report no. 1. Washington D.C.: The George Washington University, 1991.

Chickering, A., and Associates (eds.). "Learning Styles and Disciplinary Differences." *The Modern American College: Responding to the New Realities of Diverse Students and a Changing Society.* San Francisco: Jossey-Bass, 1981.

Hoeppel, J., and Wadsworth, E. (eds.). *Prevention Across the Curriculum: Curriculum Infusion for Substance Abuse Prevention in Higher Education.* Chicago: Northeastern Illinois University, 1992.

Johnson, D., Johnson, T., and Smith, K. *Cooperative Learning: Increasing College Faculty Instructional Productivity.* ASHE–ERIC Higher Education Report no. 4. Washington D.C.: The George Washington University, 1991.

Johnston, L., O'Malley, P., and Bachman, J. *Illicit Drug Use, Smoking, and Drinking by America's High School Students, College Students, and Young Adults 1975–1990.* Rockville, Md.: National Institute on Drug Abuse, 1991.

Kolb, D. *Learning Styles and Disciplinary Differences.* Chickering and Associates, 1981, p. 232–255.

Sivinicki, M. D. (ed.). *The Changing Face of College Teaching.* New Directions for Teaching and Learning, no. 42. San Francisco: Jossey-Bass, 1990.

Steinbock, C. "Drunk Driving." *Philosophy and Public Affairs,* Summer 1985, *14*, 278–295.

EMILY C. (RUSTY) WADSWORTH is associate dean of humanities at McHenry County College, Crystal Lake, Illinois.

JOHN R. HOEPPEL is director of the counseling office at Northeastern Illinois University.

R. KIPP HASSELL is dean of students at Northeastern Illinois University.

A qualitative study of five campus programs yields thirteen success factors that correlate with effective alcohol and other drug abuse prevention for students enrolled in higher education.

Characteristics of Successful Drug Prevention Programs in Higher Education

Beverly Mills-Novoa

This chapter discusses the thirteen factors found to be most critical to the success of five alcohol and other drug prevention programs in higher education in a multiple-case-study analysis of these programs. The thirteen factors are discussed in detail as well as the implications of using qualitative research methods to assess and enhance campus alcohol and other drug prevention programs. This chapter provides the context for Chapter Seven, *Striving for Success,* which presents a self-assessment tool for strengthening alcohol and other drug prevention programs in higher education.

Those who have worked with college students realize the tendency of young people, particularly in their early college years, to view the world in dualistic, simplistic terms. William Perry (1970) and others who have researched college student development have noted the importance of colleges and universities challenging students to think in more contextual, relativistic ways. As student personnel professionals, we must challenge ourselves to

The study on which this chapter is based was supported by the Fund for the Improvement of Postsecondary Education (FIPSE). I would like to thank the Northern Arizona University research team: project director Eileen V. Coughlin; technical adviser Julie Padgett; administrative assistant Jeannine Brandel; and field researchers James Fredrick, Cindy Leisse, Mary O'Neill, Jackie Twitchell-Takaki, and Phil Woodall. Additional appreciation is expressed to the five institutions that participated in this study, and to Robert Ariosto, Central Connecticut State University; R. Kipp Hassell, Northeastern Illinois University; Patricia Leonard, University of North Carolina at Wilmington; Ruth Nicholson, Valencia Community College; and Cheryl Presley, Southern Illinois University at Carbondale.

refrain from thinking in overly simplified ways about such critical topics as drug prevention. The Reagan era may have stressed that we teach students to Just Say No, but alcohol and other drug prevention in higher education is much more complex than that catch phrase implies.

In recent years, such leading authors in higher education as George Kuh, Elizabeth Whitt, and Jill Shedd (1987, p. 10) have encouraged the adoption of an emergent paradigm that acknowledges that "there is no 'real' world (i.e., single reality) to be discovered—only varied multiple realities to be individually and collectively constructed and understood." Such a paradigm shift in higher education requires that we as student personnel professionals examine our world from different vantage points.

As the previous chapters in this book indicate, alcohol and other drug prevention in higher education is a complex issue for which there are no simple or singular answers. The two-year case study research project discussed in this chapter is based on the premise that in order to understand effective alcohol and other drug prevention programs in higher education, we must first acknowledge that the contexts in which these programs function include multiple realities. This premise underlies all aspects of this research study—its design, its data analysis, and the interpretation of the data.

In September 1990, the Drug Prevention Program for the Fund for the Improvement of Postsecondary Education (FIPSE) funded Northern Arizona University in Flagstaff, Arizona, to conduct a study of five comprehensive, top-level alcohol and other drug prevention programs within institutions of higher education. This two-year evaluation study, titled *Drug Prevention Evaluation: Characteristics of Successful Programs in Higher Education,* identified the critical success factors that create and sustain successful programs.

The five institutions selected for study from the ninety-two programs funded in 1987 by FIPSE were Central Connecticut State University (New Britain), Northeastern Illinois University (Chicago), Southern Illinois University at Carbondale, the University of North Carolina at Wilmington, and Valencia Community College (Orlando, Florida). These institutions include large universities (more than 10,000 students), four-year small institutions (less than 10,000 students), two-year institutions, and both rural and urban schools. These five institutions were selected on the basis of such factors as their overall plan, campus policies, use of peer education, educational materials, special populations, organizational structure, and goal achievement. This chapter presents the process and outcomes of an in-depth look at these five institutions.

Methodology

The methodology chosen for this evaluation project was a case study design using qualitative research techniques. The researchers chose a case study design because it allowed an in-depth, qualitative look at each of the five programs. Robert K. Yin's book *Case Study Research: Design and Methods* (1989) was used as the primary reference for this study. Yin himself served as a consultant in reviewing and critiquing one of the field site reports during the second year of the project. As Yin defines it, "a case study is an empirical inquiry that investigates a contemporary phenomenon within its real-life context; when the boundaries between phenomenon and context are not clearly evident; and in which multiple sources of evidence are used" (p. 23).

To most readily and clearly understand the effectiveness of the five programs being studied, the evaluation team analyzed the programs within their institutional contexts. The case study method allowed this contextual analysis while also requiring rigorous data collection from a variety of sources and, hence, a variety of perspectives. The data sources used in this study include the review of existing documents and records; individual and group interviews; and direct observation and participation in selected campus programs, events, and the general campus environment.

The field site evaluation teams traveled in pairs and spent approximately one week at each institution included in the study. After the data from the field sites were collected and analyzed, the reports were sent back to each field site for review and comment. In addition, a round-table meeting was held at Northern Arizona University in the spring of 1992 to review the overall findings from the study with representatives from each of the field sites and a representative from FIPSE. All of these attempts to elicit feedback and to remain open to new information, perspectives, and insights enriched the study's findings and provided a series of checks and balances throughout the evaluation process.

In contrast to other studies using qualitative research techniques, this evaluation study used specific a priori propositions as an organizing factor for the study. What are a priori propositions? In this study of alcohol and other drug prevention programs in higher education, they were assumptions the researchers made before beginning the study about what factors contribute to the success of these programs. A set of propositions was developed as one of the initial steps in the study, using available research literature on successful programs to identify a preliminary list of critical success factors. These propositions were used to help determine what questions should be asked at the field sites and what data should be examined; thus, they helped to organize the study.

A *proposition,* as the *Merriam Webster Dictionary* defines it, is "2: a statement to be discussed, proved, or explained." This is very much the spirit in which propositions have been used in this study—as statements open to discussion, proof, or explanation. These propositions were revised over the course of the study as new information from each field site was uncovered. After all five field site visits were completed, the propositions were reduced to the thirteen most critical success factors. These revised propositions were then used as the basis for the development of a self-assessment tool that is currently being used by other higher education institutions as they evaluate and improve their prevention programs. This self-assessment tool is featured in Chapter Seven, "Striving for Success."

Thirteen Critical Success Factors

The thirteen factors found most critical to the success of the five alcohol and other drug prevention programs included in this case study analysis are explained below:

The program receives strong administrative support and recognition both vertically and horizontally in the institution.

Upper administrative support was a resounding theme for all five institutions. This support necessitates the active involvement of a professional in the middle to upper administrative levels who has access to top administrators at the institution and who is well-respected, influential, and credible with those administrators. These administrative advocates do not necessarily participate in the day-to-day operations of the prevention program. However, they are generally aware of current program goals and activities through a direct or indirect (but well-linked) reporting relationship with the prevention program director.

Administrative advocates tend to be creative in juggling position openings and other institutional opportunities and resources in ways that strengthen the campus drug prevention program and maintain it as a high-priority program. The support of an advocate is also visible through their active efforts to communicate prevention program activities, honors, and impact to upper administration. At Valencia Community College, for example, president Paul Gianini has been directly involved in drug prevention efforts; this top-down, hands-on support of Valencia's drug prevention program has amplified program efforts both on campus and in the community.

Successful programs also nurture support horizontally in the institution. Although all of the programs studied are organizationally located in student affairs, their relationship to academic affairs is important to institutionalization. Active networking and communication between the prevention program and other units or departments, cosponsorship of activities, and participation in departmental and institutional committees or task forces all contribute to the visibility and support of the program.

The program plans to institutionalize itself from the beginning and pursues this objective persistently.

Institutions committed to the long-term existence of a drug prevention program on campus actively plan to institutionalize the program from the day the program is started. Some grant-funded drug prevention programs, such as those funded by FIPSE, actually require an up-front commitment by each institution to continue, in some form, the drug prevention program once federal funding ceases.

Successful prevention programs, as evidenced in this study, have staff and administrators who take every opportunity to remind the institution of its need for prevention programming and its commitment to institutionalize its drug prevention program. At administrative levels, decisions are made to cement the program within the institution's organizational foundation. For example, a decision to use existing employees who are already integrated into and well-respected by the institution to staff the program increases its life expectancy. Further creation of permanent prevention positions through reorganizing when other positions open in the institution is also a step toward institutionalization.

Creating funding sources within the institution is key to the long-term financial survival of a campus alcohol and other drug prevention program. Such funding sources may be as traditional as mandatory fees for health insurance, wellness programs, or student activities. On the other hand, these sources may be creative, such as fund raising through soapbox derbies, carnivals, or selling t-shirts. Packaging successful components of the institution's drug prevention program (such as videotapes, training manuals for peers, and creative marketing ideas) and selling them to other higher education institutions, K–12 schools, or community groups is another excellent source of funds. One university has used this funding strategy by developing and selling materials regarding infusing drug prevention information into the curriculum; monies from these efforts are then used to bolster drug prevention efforts on their own campus. Identifying alumni willing to provide endowments for drug prevention efforts is an additional creative funding strategy that provides tax benefits and personal satisfaction to the alumni while providing an independent source of funding.

The program affects institutional regulations regarding alcohol and other drug use through policy formation, communication, and enforcement.

Because policies and their implementation remain an integral part of organizational life in higher education, successful prevention programs appropriately link themselves with the formation, communication, and implementation of policies on campus, especially those concerned with institutional alcohol and other drug use. The guidelines created by the Network of Colleges and Universities Committee for the Elimination of Drug and Alcohol Abuse can serve as a reference point for such policy formation and implementation.

Through strong linkages between the drug prevention program and institutional regulations, the program is further woven into the organizational fabric of the institution and serves an integral function. This is critically important because institutional values are stated in the rules regarding alcohol and other drug use. In all the institutions studied, the campus drug prevention program plays a significant role in the communication and interpretation of campus policies regarding alcohol and other drugs. At the University of North Carolina at Wilmington, for example, the staff for the campus drug prevention program took a large role in the development of a thorough *Substance Abuse Handbook* for faculty, staff, and students that includes institutional policies on alcohol, illegal drugs, penalties, and the referral process for students. Often the program staff is actively involved in raising interpretive issues regarding policies and advising others in the institution regarding these issues.

The prevention programs studied also influence institutional policy by questioning campus support for activities that condone substance abuse (such as traditional campus festivals centered around alcohol, alcohol-related sponsorship of athletic events, the marketing or advertising of alcoholic beverages on campus, and tailgate parties).

Prevention programs also receive visibility through their link with drug-related policies. Campus alcohol and other drug prevention programs are often touted both on and off campus as the institution's serious response to substance abuse at each institution. In one institution, the presence of the campus drug prevention program helps to relieve town–gown tensions caused by student parties held in the community. That program features a series of required educational seminars for students who violate the institution's alcohol policy. In this way, the drug prevention program is able to reinforce the institution's drug policies while providing education and insight to student offenders.

The program targets ways to encourage individuals to personalize substance abuse issues and involves many campus groups, creating a ripple effect.

The five drug prevention programs studied also have built campuswide support for their efforts by emphasizing the personalization of drug prevention issues. Such personalization attempts are evident in presentation titles ("You Booze and Cruise and We All Lose! DWI Facts") as well as activities focused on getting students, staff, and faculty personally in touch with the impact of drug use and abuse. Central Connecticut State University organized a wall of commitment on which students, staff, and faculty could indicate their personal commitments for reducing alcohol and other drug problems.

A number of the programs studied feature student, faculty, and staff training on how to intervene with a friend, family member, or co-worker with an alcohol or other drug problem. Such training is popular on campus because it enables individuals to actually do something when confronted with these issues in their own lives. By getting individuals to personalize the effects of drug abuse and to identify actions that could be taken to prevent drug abuse, the successful programs are able to encourage psychological ownership of the prevention program, its vision, and its strategies across campus. This, in turn, creates a ripple effect within the institution.

The program creates a strong marketing approach for publicizing the program, its activities, positive role models, and prevention messages.

The prevention programs included in this case study analysis recognize the importance of vigorously marketing the prevention program and its activities on campus to achieve high visibility. A number of the programs studied, especially those with higher numbers of residential students or that have a campus-centered student population use a broad range of marketing techniques to raise on-campus visibility. These marketing techniques include advertisements, brochures, newsletters, newspaper columns, displays, and attention-getting campuswide activities.

Southern Illinois University at Carbondale, for example, features a "Dr. Buzz" newspaper advice column for "Advice to the Drug-Worn" that appears in a campus newspaper that has extensive readership on campus and in the community. The column provides factual yet sensitive and personal responses to such questions as, "If I keep drinking even though I know I'm already drunk, could that mean I might be in danger of becoming an alcoholic?"

Another campus prevention program, the University of North Carolina at Wilmington, features a special newsletter called *Highlites* to serve as a communication vehicle from the program to the campus community. This newsletter, coordinated and produced by a peer educator, presents drug-related issues, health tips, drug-related videotapes available through the program, and advertisements for program events.

Even the titles for educational events are catchy and inviting. For example, one campus holds "RAD" educational sessions and advertises them by asking "Are you RAD (Rethinking About Drinking)?" Another campus sponsors presentations titled "Sizzlin' Love Triangles: You, Your Date, and Booze," "Acids, 'Shrooms, and Ecstacy," and "Of Lites, Silver Bullets, Bulls, and Heineys" (featuring information on common alcoholic beverages, their contents, effects, and marketing). All of these means of attracting student audiences are ways to market the prevention program and its educational prevention messages.

The program capitalizes on local, state, and federal visibility and recognition for program excellence to increase immunity to institutional budget cuts.

Successful drug prevention programs capitalize on program visibility gained at local, state, or national levels in recognition of program or outreach efforts. Such visibility may result from staff involvement in local, state, or national drug prevention efforts (such as the Network of Colleges and Universities Committee for the Elimination of Drug and Alcohol Abuse, local substance abuse agency boards, and governor's drug prevention efforts) or through additional grant involvement (such as FIPSE dissemination or consortium grants, Department of Education Drug Free Schools Grants for Teacher Education, and Community Assistance Grants). Even being selected as one of the field sites for this national study of drug prevention programs was cited by each of the five institutions as a boon to program prestige within their institutions and in the surrounding communities.

Some successful prevention programs attain visibility through achieving awards for their on-campus efforts (such as National Drug Awareness Week competitions) and by having program staff and others on campus do local and national presentations, give radio and television interviews, or write articles. Cosponsorship with the community for selected awareness activities such as drug awareness fairs and national speakers also markets the prevention program externally while stretching its resource dollars.

Gaining a local, state, or national reputation for program excellence not only gives the prevention program visibility but adds to its immunity to program cuts because it is viewed publicly as a winner. This is one benefit successful programs receive from marketing their program and its accomplishments to upper-level administrators and trustees via memos, meeting updates, campus and local newspaper articles, and personal communication. In this way, they capitalize on the high visibility of their exemplary program and outreach efforts.

The program selects program staff for diversity of skills, strong community ties, broad-based expertise in prevention education with special expertise in substance abuse, excellent communication skills, personal compatibility, enthusiasm, and dedicated, persistent commitment.

Unequivocally, all five institutions with successful programs included in this study emphasize high-quality staff as a critical success factor. Important staff competencies include the following:

Knowledge and Skills
  Up-to-date knowledge regarding substance abuse
  Good communication skills
  Marketing knowledge and skills
  Teaching and facilitating skills
  Political astuteness and active on- and off-campus networks
  Knowledge of organization development and change management
  Ability to work creatively with limited budget and time constraints
  Ability to see parts in relation to the whole
Personal Characteristics
  Commitment and dedication to the program vision
  Creativity and high energy
  Willingness to try new things and take risks
  Persistence and resilience, including the ability to deal with resistance and failures)
  Collaborative attitude

Flexibility and openness to other people's ideas, including students' ideas
Ability to build credibility with faculty
Sensitivity to student issues
Self-confidence and self-assuredness
Sense of humor and ability to have fun
Ability to maintain balance between work and personal life

Certainly, individual staff do not possess all of these competencies, but, in general, they complement each others' areas of competence. All of the case studies emphasize the project staff as the linchpin for the program's success.

The program promotes an institutional environment that supports no use for students under legal age, with an emphasis on responsible, personal decision making; the program also stresses a nonjudgmental, positive, fact-based approach in disseminating information.

Institutions in this case study analysis already had a policy in place before the inception of their drug prevention programs. These policies uniformly specified no use for students under twenty-one.

Legally, higher education institutions cannot condone, promote, or otherwise encourage alcohol use by students under the legal drinking age of twenty-one. Concern in recent years regarding the potential legal liability of colleges and universities and organizations such as fraternities, sororities, and other student groups for alcohol-related accidents and fatalities has added strength to the rationale for no-use policies for underage students. The methods by which these policies are enforced, however, is a different matter.

The institutions included in this study generally try to keep an open line of communication between campus police, the dean of students or other disciplinary administrative offices, and the alcohol and other drug prevention program. The University of North Carolina at Wilmington, for example, has campus police representation on its drug prevention program advisory committee and uses campus police in selected campus presentations. The alcohol and other drug prevention program at this institution reports to the dean of students, who is actively involved in its support and programming. Such communication allows the issue of policy enforcement to emerge in a constructive tone and promotes a teamwork approach in addressing prevention, policy enforcement, and consequences.

Despite an institution's legal responsibilities and policy enforcement efforts, the reality of college life is that a large number of its student population, whether of legal age or not, will choose to drink. The programs included in this study respond to that reality by rejecting a simplistic "Just Say No" approach. These programs instead recognize the importance of promoting individual responsibility and decision making among their emerging adult students.

As a result, noncomplicated alcohol violations are most often responded to with discussions with RAs, letters of warning, and educational approaches that encourage students to make positive choices. Multiple violations or violations that include other behavioral issues are most often responded to with greater disciplinary action.

Successful prevention programs focus on providing students with accurate information regarding alcohol and other drugs in a nonjudgmental way that acknowledges the individual's responsibility for making decisions regarding alcohol and other drug use. Such approaches do not negate the institution's legal responsibilities regarding *no use* policies for underage students, but recognize that students of all ages have and will continue to make decisions about their drinking behavior—whether to drink, when to drink, how much to drink, with whom and under what circumstances.

One method used at Central Connecticut State University to promote an institutional environment that supports effective individual decision making regarding alcohol is a life-style risk reduction approach, the On-Campus Talking About Alcohol program (OCTAA) developed by the Prevention Research Institute in Lexington, Kentucky. This approach emphasizes research-based presentations to aid individuals in their personal decisions about alcohol use in their lives.

Responsible decision making in the prevention program studied is promoted through a positive, upbeat, nonjudgmental tone. These programs emphasize fact-based handouts that feature information such as body weight charts and alcohol concentration data. Presentations, workshops, and materials are relatively free of moralistic messages and instead emphasize facts and potential consequences.

The program ties alcohol and other drug use to the impact on personal health, self-esteem, and wellness, promotes activities that reinforce the positive, drug-free elements of student life, and emphasizes alternative activities and natural highs.

Wellness has become a popular vessel for prevention. The emphasis on wellness allows programs latitude to talk about lifestyle choices and physical and mental health. Wellness is generally viewed as a positive theme and helps to offset the negative tone often associated with discussing alcohol and other drug abuse. In the wellness context, alcohol and other drug decisions are reframed as healthy or unhealthy life-style choices.

In addition, successful prevention programs recognize the linkage between alcohol and other drugs and related issues such as stress, acquaintance rape, and low self-esteem. As a result, they provide programming that aids students in exploring alternative ways of dealing with these issues (such as more effective ways of reducing stress, achieving social acceptance, and making informed sexual decisions). Through an understanding of the issues that concern students, prevention programs can focus on strategies linked to these issues. Such linkages provide a broader context for presenting prevention issues on campus.

Emphasis on alcohol-free recreational activities, or natural highs, is a positive reframing of the campus environment. At the University of North Carolina at Wilmington, a program titled *Alternatives!* emphasizes this approach. *Alternatives!* sponsors numerous alcohol-free activities for students (e.g., rope course trips, whitewater rafting, camping, and canoeing adventures). Another prevention program at Central Connecticut State University served as an advocate for building a campuswide, year-round recreational facility. This facility features athletic opportunities such as tennis courts and a running track that provide alternative alcohol-free recreation for students.

The program demonstrates a clear understanding of the special needs of the institution and its culturally diverse student population and finds prevention strategies to fit the campus.

Successful drug prevention programs are in tune with their campus, its culture, and its distinctive personality. They emphasize drug prevention strategies that are sensitive to their students' needs and characteristics. Campuses with high numbers of commuter students, for example, focus on affecting the staff and faculty because they are the common denominator and chief influence for the drop-in, drop-out commuter population.

The three commuter institutions studied, Northeastern Illinois University, Valencia Community College, and Central Connecticut State University, rely on the infusion of drug prevention education modules into the academic curriculum as their primary prevention strategy. Commuter campuses have found that the process of writing the prevention education modules increases awareness of alcohol and other drug issues among faculty members. The process of educating faculty about integrating the modules into the curriculum exposes faculty to alcohol and other drug information and demonstrates how the material applies to their particular subject area. Once this connection is clear, faculty excitement and involvement increase and faculty become interested in conducting prevention-related research and projects on their own (such as a critique of codependency from a feminist perspective, or coediting of a book on substance abuse).

Central Connecticut State University created a Student Assistance Program (SAP) as a primary prevention program strategy. Through the SAP, selected staff and faculty are trained to assist students on a wide range of problems including alcohol use and abuse, friends or family who abuse alcohol or other drugs, relationship issues, self-esteem issues, and family difficulties. This responsive program's ability to deal with multiple personal problems, with special emphasis on substance abuse issues, provides a safety net for its commuter students.

The two other institutions included in the case study analysis, Southern Illinois University at Carbondale and the University of North Carolina at Wilmington, feature predominantly residential or close to campus student populations. Because residential or campus-centered institutions tend to have students on campus longer and in more predictable patterns, they emphasize working with and through students to achieve program goals and activities. In these programs, peer educators are the primary force behind the development and implementation of program activities. The use of peer educators enables these programs to maintain a strong student perspective in their activities and events. These programs put extensive effort into selecting and training peer educators to serve as activity developers, coordinators, educators, and role models.

The prevention activities at student-oriented campuses are extremely varied and creative. Examples include mocktails (cocktails without alcohol), health fairs, debates, "Think Smart" programs in which prison inmates talk about their experiences with drugs, special holiday events (such as a "Say Booo to Drugs" theme at Halloween), and classroom presentations. These student-oriented programs take advantage of the captive audiences in residence halls, Greek fraternities and sororities, and athletic teams to institute ongoing programming that is generally implemented by student educators.

A common theme in prevention programs is sensitivity to campus culture and institutional peculiarities in designing drug prevention strategies. Although each campus generally implements multiple strategies (such as curriculum infusion efforts, student educator groups, educational programming for residence halls and athletes, and student assistance programs), there are generally one or, at the most, two major strategies that become keystone activities for the prevention program. Focusing on one or two strategies initially that fit the campus environment and implementing those strategies well seems to yield better results than a shotgun approach in which a little is done in a lot of areas with no real focus.

The program uses a needs assessment as a first step to detail alcohol and other drug-related problems or issues (such as acquaintance rape, vandalism, stress) and to identify what resources exist on and off campus to address these issues.

The successful drug-prevention programs studied emphasize an initial assessment of drug-related issues and resources at the institution. They also continue to monitor those needs, issues, and resources over time after establishing an initial baseline. All of the programs studied use assessment surveys to monitor the campus pulse regarding substance abuse issues, attitudes, and usage. These assessments consist of campus surveys, focus groups, or individual interviews with students, faculty, and administrators. Generally, these occur on a periodic basis and provide insight into immediate campus concerns and needs. One program, for example, identified stress, overeating, and Adult Children of Alcoholics (ACOA) issues through its assessment survey and, subsequently, realigned its campus programming to address these needs.

The program is allied organizationally with a department or center that adds credibility to its efforts, promotes a positive image, and contributes information and resources.

Successful prevention programs, in general, can be characterized as campuswide programs from their inception. This shared ownership approach stresses the involvement of an expanding network of people from as many key areas of campus as possible.

A common organizational success factor is strong alliances with departments and centers that add credibility to prevention efforts. Although actual affiliations differ from program to program (for example, the program may be part of a Wellness Center or a separate program under the dean of students), the program must fit comfortably under that unit's mission, be positioned as a positive, not punitive function, and benefit from the relationships, resources, information, and reputation provided by that department. This is not to say that some prevention programs do not have educational activities focused on alcohol-related student disciplinary cases, but that such functions are only a small part of the prevention program and do not overshadow the upbeat, educational tone of the program. At the University of North Carolina at Wilmington, for example, the drug prevention program reports to the dean of students and does conduct educational sessions for student alcohol and other drug policy offenders, but such activities are only a small part of the prevention program's emphasis on providing alcohol-free recreational activities and natural highs for students.

The program is based on a sound planning process and reviews and evaluates its efforts on a regular basis.

As organizational units, successful prevention programs generally use strategic planning techniques in which goals are set and progress is periodically evaluated. In turn, project staff allow time for collective reflection so that the program and its strategies and activities can be evaluated and refocused to reflect changing campus needs.

Successful programs also use evaluation strategies to monitor program effectiveness. Such strategies typically include questionnaires after workshops or educational sessions and pre- and post-surveys after an educational series or curriculum infusion module. In addition, a campus might also use a process consultation and evaluation model in which an outside evaluator meets regularly with project staff to discuss evaluation strategies and activities.

Southern Illinois University at Carbondale creatively met its evaluation needs by providing research opportunities for graduate students. At this campus, two master's degree students designed extensive evaluation plans for the program materials and the knowledge, attitude, and behavior of program participants as part of their thesis work. In addition, a doctoral candidate at that campus developed an evaluation design and procedures for evaluating the program's peer training program. This campus has been able to provide valuable real-life learning opportunities for its graduate students while gleaning invaluable data regarding the effectiveness of program components.

Conclusions

At each of the five institutions included in this case study analysis, the researchers examined each campus and prevention program from a variety of perspectives. The qualitative research methods used provided the researchers with a sense of the multiple realities that make up each campus and, hence, the context for each campus drug prevention program.

In some cases, looking at these prevention programs from multiple perspectives merely confirmed our original assumptions or a priori propositions. Such confirmation can itself be useful as it reinforces what a program is doing right and clarifies those specific success factors. For example, as researchers, we would have surmised that successful alcohol and other drug prevention programs are, from an organizational standpoint, well-run, well-planned, and well-implemented programs with both vertical and horizontal networks of support throughout the institution. What we would not have necessarily seen before examining the five campuses was the importance of having administrative advocates, top administrators who communicate program activities and accomplishments upward in the organization and actively seek ways to organizationally strengthen the prevention program.

In turn, had we not visited several sites and gained a variety of perspectives at each site, we would not have fully understood the importance of each prevention program having a firm grasp of the special needs of the institution and its student population. During the course of this two-year study, it became clear that there is no one-size-fits-all prevention program approach for higher education institutions. In fact, successful alcohol and other drug prevention programs, as reflected in our analysis, have a keen grasp of the multiple realities of which their campuses are composed and develop prevention strategies that are tailored to those campuses and diverse student populations.

By using qualitative research methods, the research team was able to see effective drug prevention in higher education from a richer, contextual perspective. Through the use of the self-assessment tool included in the last chapter of this book, or through the use of other qualitatively based tools, each higher education institution can begin to view its own prevention program from a different perspective—a perspective that recognizes the multiple realities of campus life.

References

Kuh, G. D., Whitt, E. J., and Shedd, J. D. *Student Affairs Work, 2001: A Paradigmatic Odyssey.* Alexandria, Va.: American College Personnel Association, 1987, p. 10.

Perry, W. G., Jr. *Forms of Intellectual and Ethical Development in the College Years.* New York: Holt, Rinehart & Winston, 1970.

Yin, R. K. *Case Study Research: Design and Methods.* Newbury Park, Calif.: Sage, 1989, p. 23.

BEVERLY MILLS-NOVOA is a partner in Mills-Novoa and Associates, a human resource consulting firm specializing in balancing work and family issues and qualitative evaluation research.

Comprehensive prevention programs need a benchmark for success. Self-assessment based on characteristics of successful programs provides a strategic planning method, evaluation tool, and the needed benchmark.

Striving for Success

Beverly Mills-Novoa, Eileen V. Coughlin

An important component of effecting campuswide change is self-assessment. The self-assessment tool featured in this chapter encourages college campuses to look at the success factors needed to undergird alcohol and other drug prevention programs in higher education. It can be used in a variety of ways at any point in the campuswide drug prevention change process—whether prevention efforts are just beginning or have been in place for some time.

Often self-assessment is lumped in the category of evaluation—a seemingly after-the-fact examination of what has been done to affect drug-related attitudes and behaviors on campus. In reality, good program self-assessment is a proactive form of evaluation that occurs before, during, and after prevention efforts are in place. It allows periodic snapshots of the campus during the change process and feeds back information that can help drug prevention efforts to come increasingly in focus and on target.

Background and Purpose of the Tool

The self-assessment tool is based on the characteristics of successful programs identified in the drug prevention evaluation study presented in Chapter Six. The researchers spent approximately one week at each of five selected field site institutions examining existing documents, conducting in-depth interviews, and observing and participating in prevention-related activities. The use of these qualitative research methods allowed Northern Arizona University's research team to gather rich, in-depth information that has practical application in strategic planning and program assessment. However, these factors are intended to remain flexible and should be used selectively with an openness to changing data and institutional context. Collection of data that test the efficacy of these critical factors on your campus is encouraged.

New Directions for Student Services, no. 67, Fall 1994 © Jossey-Bass Publishers

The assessment guide is a qualitative benchmark for both planning and evaluation of prevention programs. It is intended to aid top administrators in developing strategic plans for new prevention efforts as well as providing guidelines for practitioners in the improvement and continued success of their programs.

Use of the Self-Assessment Guide for Strategic Planning

The self-assessment guide can aid administrators in developing strategic plans for an institutional alcohol and other drug prevention program. The thirteen critical success factors provide clues on organizational structure, funding plans, policy development, hiring, and selection of staff. A quick review and rating of these critical factors, done individually or in group settings, ensures that future planning efforts take into account factors that affect the success of prevention programs.

A more in-depth look at each of the thirteen factors as they relate to a specific institution's prevention program will yield even greater information. This in-depth study might also be used in conjunction with an SWOT process. In this application, each characteristic would be reviewed in terms of the Strengths, Weaknesses, Opportunities, and Threats of current programs within each of the thirteen success factors. The outcome of this process would allow the institution to build on existing strengths.

Use of the Self-Assessment Guide for Program Improvement

The self-assessment guide can also be used by alcohol and other drug prevention practitioners to improve delivery of services. Careful review and rating of the thirteen critical factors provide focus and effective use of resources. Training and professional development can be designed around the staff competencies needed to improve the success of the prevention program. Staff evaluations can also include measurements of progress within the thirteen areas.

You may want to make copies of the blank forms throughout the guide for use by colleagues during the assessment and planning process.

Critical Success Factors

The reports from the five individual field sites were reviewed extensively to determine cross-institutional findings and general patterns applicable to other higher education institutions as they plan for and improve their prevention programs. This extensive review yielded thirteen factors critical to the success of alcohol and other drug prevention programs in higher education. Figure 7.1 underscores the importance of these factors, in concert with the alcohol and other drug prevention program and campus culture, in yielding program success.

Figure 7.1. The Elements of Program Success

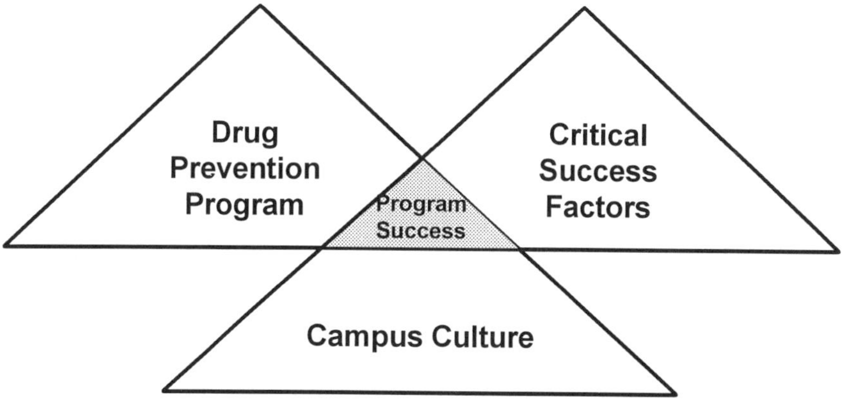

The Critical Success Factors in Context

The thirteen factors that were found to contribute to the success of five diverse prevention programs in higher education are described in Chapter Six, *Characteristics of Successful Drug Prevention Programs in Higher Education,* to aid you in using the self-assessment tools provided in this guide. The explanations furnished in Chapter Six provide a context for understanding the thirteen critical success factors.

Other Assessment Methods

In addition to this qualitative assessment of your efforts, use of quantitative longitudinal student use data is encouraged. Participation in the Core instrument data collection is one possible approach to data collection that allows national and regional comparisons. Quantitative data on student use must be viewed in terms of the changing context of and use in society. Measures of success on an individual campus should be evaluated on a cohort basis to ensure that reported use is from students who have had the opportunity to be affected by the campus prevention efforts. For this reason, some campuses may want to collect use data on subpopulations of students who can be followed over the course of four to five years.

Final Thoughts

Assessing prevention efforts requires evaluating what did *not* happen. Prevention is an attempt to obstruct or impede the progress of undesirable behavior. Hence, the very connotation of the word *prevention* may hamper self-assessment and data collection. This not only restricts our ability to assess, but also may narrow our view of the possibilities. We are often so focused on what we *don't* want to happen that we fail to view drug prevention as something positive and tangible. This volume has presented a number of ideas to help student services professionals view drug prevention from a variety of vantage points and positive perspectives. In the final analysis, the vital question is not what we hope to prevent, but rather what we hope to create that will make a difference in drug prevention efforts in higher education.

Appendix: Success Factor Planning Worksheet, Rating Form, and Action Planning Worksheet

The purpose of the Planning Worksheet and the Rating Form is to provide prevention practitioners in higher education with a tool for improving and further developing their existing programs. The purpose of the Action Planning Worksheet is to aid you and your colleagues in targeting your institution's prevention program needs and putting together action plans for strengthening your program. Completion of these forms requires an in-depth analysis of all or selected critical success factors in your prevention program. This intensive review of the prevention program can lead to plans for maintaining current program strengths and addressing program needs.

To complete the Planning Worksheet and the Rating Form, complete the following steps:

1. *Read completely through the information provided on each critical success factor discussed in Chapter Six.*

Review the thirteen success factors. Think about how each factor relates to your institution's prevention program. You may want to do a preliminary rating of the thirteen factors for your program using the Rating Form (Exhibit 7.2) and then investigate selected success factors about which there is disagreement among you and your colleagues or that are generally perceived as untrue for your institution's prevention program. Another alternative for using the Planning Worksheet and the Rating Form is to investigate all thirteen factors as they relate to your institution's prevention program.

2. *Brainstorm, by yourself or with colleagues, a list of questions that relate to each success factor being reviewed.*

For example, in reviewing the first success factor, "The program receives strong administrative support and recognition both vertically and horizontally in the institution," sample questions you might develop include the following:

- To what extent have our upper-level administrators committed to the long-term continuation of the program?
- How do our top administrators demonstrate their support of the program?
- What recognition has the program received from top administration?
- How is information about the program communicated to senior administrators? To other units within the institution?

- How does the prevention staff relate to other units in the institution? Do they participate in cross-departmental committees or task forces or cosponsor activities? Is there informal, ongoing communication with staff from various units?

These questions can be noted on the Planning Worksheet (Exhibit 7.1) under the Key Questions column.

Directions: Note key questions you or your colleagues have brainstormed for each critical success factor targeted for further investigation in your prevention program. Determine the most appropriate information sources for getting answers to the list of key questions developed for each success factor under review.

3. *Determine the most appropriate information sources for answers to the list of key questions you developed for each success factor under review. Those information sources might include the following:*

- Existing documents, such as minutes of meetings, annual reports, memos, or evaluation data.
- Individual or group interviews with people associated with the program such as the president, vice presidents, program directors (including those from other units), program staff and their colleagues in other units, faculty, and students (both those involved in program activities and others interviewed randomly on campus).
- Observation and participation in program activities and events.

These data sources can be noted for each respective success factor on the Planning Worksheet (Exhibit 7.1) under the Information Sources column.

4. *Determine and implement a realistic plan for gathering such information in a cost-effective manner.*

You may find that the actual process of gathering such data not only is enlightening and insightful but produces increased ownership in the prevention program itself by eliciting participation in the review process across the campus.

5. *Rate each success factor being reviewed in terms of how characteristic it is of your institution's prevention program.*

Use the information gathered in steps 2 through 4 as the basis for your rating. Using the Rating Form (Exhibit 7.2), record these ratings.

Directions: Read the explanation of each success factor provided in Chapter Six. Note below the degree to which each factor is characteristic of your prevention program based on a review of existing documents, interviews, focus groups, and observations regarding your program. Use the rating scale from 1 to 5 provided below to note how characteristic a factor is of your institution's prevention program.

Exhibit 7.1. Planning Worksheet

Critical Success Factors	Key Questions	Information Sources
(1) Strong administrative support		
(2) Institutionalization of program		
(3) Policy impact		
(4) Personalization of issues/ripple effect on campus		
(5) Strong marketing approach		
(6) Local, state, or federal recognition		
(7) Program staff with diverse skills		
(8) Emphasis on responsible, personal decision making and non judgmental, positive, fact-based program approach		
(9) Tie to personal health, self-esteem, wellness, and emphasis on alternative activities		
(10) Prevention strategies that fit the campus		
(11) Use of needs assessment		
(12) Organizational alliance with department or center that lends credibility and promotes a positive image		
(13) Sound planning and evaluation processes		

Exhibit 7.2. Rating Form

How well does this success factor characterize your drug prevention program?

Not at All	Not Very	Somewhat	Generally	Most
1	2	3	4	5

____ (1)   Receives strong administrative support and recognition both verically and horizontally in the institution.

____ (2)   Plans to institutionalize the program from the beginning and pursues this objective persistently.

____ (3)   Affects institutional rules and regulations regarding alcohol and other drug use through policy formation, communication, and enforcement.

____ (4)   Targets ways to encourage individuals to personalize substance abuse issues and involves multiple campus groups in creating a ripple effect on campus.

____ (5)   Creates a strong marketing approach for publicizing the program, its activities, positive role models and prevention messages.

____ (6)   Capitalizes on local, state, or federal visibility and recognition for program excellence to increase immunity to institutional budget cuts.

____ (7)   Selects program staff for diversity of skills, strong community ties, broad-based experise in prevention education with special expertise in substance abuse, excellent communication skills, personal compatibility, enthusiasm, and dedicated, persistent commitment.

____ (8)   Promotes an institutional environment that supports no use for students under legal age, with an emphasis on responsible, personal decision making; the program also stresses a nonjudgmental positive, fact-based tone and approach in disseminating prevention information.

____ (9)   Ties alcohol and other drug use to the impact on personal health, self-esteem aand wellness; promotes activities that reinforce the positive, drug-free element of student life and emphasizes alternative activities and natural highs.

____ (10) Demonstrates a clear understanding of the special needs of the institution and its culturally diverse student population and finds prevention strategies to fit the campus.

____ (11) Uses a needs assessment as a first step to detail alcohol and other drug-related problems (acquaintance rape, vandalism, stress) and to identify what resources exist on and off campus to address these issues.

____ (12) Is allied organizationally with a department or center that lends credibility to its efforts, promotes a positive image, and contributes information and resources.

____ (13) Bases its prog.rams on a sound planning process and reviews and evaluates program efforts regularly.

6. *Refer to the Action Planning Worksheet (Exhibit 7.3). This worksheet focuses on developing a plan for maintaining program strengths and targeting areas where improvement is needed in your alcohol and other prevention program.*

The purpose of this worksheet (Exhibit 7.3) is to aid you and your colleagues in targeting your institution's prevention program needs and putting together action plans for strengthening your program.

Directions: To complete the Action Planning Worksheet complete the following steps:

1. Review the Planning Worksheet (Exhibit 7.1) and Rating Form (Exhibit 7.2).
2. Determine your prevention program's needs according to your findings from the Rating Form (the success factors that were rated a 1 or 2).
3. List up to five program needs on the Action Planning Worksheet (Exhibit 7.3). If your institution has more than five needs, select the five that, according to your best judgment or that of your colleagues, are most important for program success in your specific institution.
4. Develop plans for strengthening these success factors. Note these plans in the space provided below the five program needs on the Action Planning Worksheet. You may wish to use additional sheets of paper to fully document your plans for addressing your program's needs.

Exhibit 7.3. Action Planning Worksheet

Program Needs	1.
	2.
	3.
	4.
	5.
Action Plans	*Plans for strengthening these success factors in your institution's drug prevention program:*

Reference

Mills-Novoa, B. *Striving for Success: A Self-Assessment Guide for Strengthening Drug Prevention Programs in Higher Education.* Flagstaff: Northern Arizona University, August 1992.

BEVERLY MILLS-NOVOA is a partner in Mills-Novoa and Associates, a human resource consulting firm specializing in balancing work and family issues and qualitative evaluation research.

EILEEN V. COUGHLIN is vice president for student affairs/dean for academic support services at Western Washington University, Bellingham. She was also director of the qualitative evaluation project presented in Chapter Six.

As we look to the future, higher education must continue to
develop multiple strategies with an ear to the voice of our students
and an eye to the mirror image reflected by the data.

Conclusions and Resources

Eileen V. Coughlin

The intent of this volume is, in part, to provide an opportunity to explore our professional attitudes and resulting contributions in the area of alcohol and other drug prevention in student affairs. Presley, Meilman, and Padgett have armed us with the facts and myths. Leonard and Edwards have provided the theoretical understanding of student culture with particular tips on recreating culture through students as change agents. Mills-Novoa and Coughlin have contributed a new assessment tool based on characteristics of success. Wadsworth, Hoeppel, and Hassell have presented a curriculum infusion model that is particularly useful for community colleges and commuter campuses, and Gianini and Nicholson have provided tips on how to gain presidential support. These authors have provided some of the right answers. The hope is that their work will stimulate additional advances in eliminating the ghost of NOT ME.

There is an old Chinese proverb that is relevant to our continued progress in alcohol and drug prevention. "One disease, long life; no disease, short life" (Hoff, 1985, p. 48). If we can name the disease, it is possible to prevent its destructive influence. However, if we continue to assert that there is no disease, instead of living happily ever after we will live happily after ever.

Students themselves have identified significant deleterious effects of illicit drug use and alcohol abuse. Their voice is heard in both the quantitative data and in their anecdotes. Thirty-two percent of the students included in the Core instrument indicated that they missed class in the previous year due to alcohol abuse. However, only 7 percent indicated involvement in active prevention efforts. Our challenge is to reverse these two figures through multiple strategies that match appropriate prevention to the personal context each student brings to higher education.

Alcohol and other drug prevention in higher education must sustain intense programming because the entire student population is regenerated every five to six years. In order to accept this challenge, higher education must accept its weakness. Perhaps Ernest Boyer said it best: "All human communities have their dark side, and college communities are no exception . . . the same environment that fosters personal growth, learning, and commitment to others may also intensify the dangers of drug and alcohol abuse" (Rivinus, 1988, p. xi). Throughout this book, we have emphasized a holistic perspective in addressing drug prevention efforts on campus. This inclusive view is intended to encourage us, as administrators and practitioners, to examine our campuses systematically and to choose multiple entry points for drug prevention efforts.

Clearly, the creation of a healthy campus climate requires collective efforts. There is no better profession to lead this endeavor than student affairs. Our experience in facilitating the development of community is the hallmark of our profession. The following resource list is offered as additional support in broadening our understanding of campus prevention efforts.

Books

Rivinus, T. M. (ed.). *Alcoholism/Chemical Dependency and the College Student.* New York: Haworth, 1988.

This book provides both counseling and administrative perspectives on education and treatment of college students. It provides an excellent overview of issues including working with adult children of alcoholics, theoretical perspectives, and the prevention education issues.

Lawson, G. W., and Lawson, A. W. (eds.). *Alcoholism and Substance Abuse in Special Populations.* Rockville, Md.: Aspen, 1989.

Lawson and Lawson's book is an excellent reference on special populations of abusers including Hispanics, Native Americans, gay men and lesbians, the disabled, and women. This work is not specifically focused on students, but does provide some insight into specialized issues of subpopulations.

Longitudinal Research

Johnston, L. D., O'Malley, P. M., and Bachman, J. G. *National Survey Results on Drug Uses from Monitoring the Future Student 1975–1992 Volume 1 (Secondary School Students) and Volume 2 (College Students and Young Adults).* Rockville, Md.: National Institutes of Health, 1993.

The ongoing study conducted by the University of Michigan Institute for Social Research is one of the best sources of data on student alcohol and other drug use. It includes a broad spectrum of drug use from cigarettes to heroin. The sampling includes eighth, tenth, and twelfth graders as well as college students. This work is invaluable for anticipating future college student use.

Presley, C. A., Meilman, P. W., and Lyerla, R. *Alcohol and Drugs on American College Campuses: Use, Consequences, and Perceptions of the Campus Environment, Vol. I, 1989–91.* Carbondale: Southern Illinois University, 1993.

This research includes college students' responses to an instrument that was developed in 1989 by representatives from institutions of higher education across the country. This work includes use and consequences data and provides some interesting geographical and type-of-institution data that are useful for benchmarking.

Other Works

Goodale, T. G. *I Thought I Could Handle Alcohol and Drug Abuse.* Washington, D.C.: Association of Governing Boards of Universities and Colleges, 1992.

This monograph is succinct and includes an overview of abuse issues on American college campuses as well as a focus on governing boards' role in supporting prevention and intervention on the college campus.

Gehring, D. D., and Geraci, C. P. *Alcohol on Campus: A Compendium of the Law and A Guide to Campus Policy.* Asheville, N.C.: College Administration Publications, 1989.

This is the best source I have found on a comprehensive review of the law and sources of liability for campus. It includes explanations of types of liability along with a state-by-state inclusive review of case law affecting higher education.

References

Hoff, B. *The Tao of Pooh.* New York: Penguin, 1985, p. 48.
Rivinus, T. M. *Alcoholism/Chemical Dependency and the College Student.* New York: Haworth, 1988, p. xi.

EILEEN V. COUGHLIN is vice president for student affairs/dean for academic support services at Western Washington University, Bellingham. She was also director of the qualitative evaluation project presented in Chapters Six and Seven.

INDEX

ORDERING INFORMATION

NEW DIRECTIONS FOR STUDENT SERVICES is a series of paperback books that offers guidelines and programs for aiding students in their total development—emotional, social, and physical, as well as intellectual. Books in the series are published quarterly in spring, summer, fall, and winter and are available for purchase by subscription as well as by single copy.

SUBSCRIPTIONS for 1994 cost $47.00 for individuals (a savings of 25 percent over single-copy prices) and $62.00 for institutions, agencies, and libraries. Please do not send institutional checks for personal subscriptions. Standing orders are accepted.

SINGLE COPIES cost $15.95 when payment accompanies order. (California, New Jersey, New York, and Washington, D.C., residents please include appropriate sales tax.) Billed orders will be charged postage and handling.

DISCOUNTS FOR QUANTITY ORDERS are available. Please write to the address below for information.

ALL ORDERS must include either the name of an individual or an official purchase order number. Please submit your order as follows:
    Subscriptions: specify series and year subscription is to begin
    Single copies: include individual title code (such as SS55)

MAIL ALL ORDERS TO:
    Jossey-Bass Publishers
    350 Sansome Street
    San Francisco, California 94104-1342

FOR SUBSCRIPTION SALES OUTSIDE OF THE UNITED STATES, CONTACT:
    any international subscription agency or Jossey-Bass directly.

OTHER TITLES AVAILABLE IN THE
NEW DIRECTIONS FOR STUDENT SERVICES SERIES
Margaret J. Barr, Editor-in-Chief
M. Lee Upcraft, Associate Editor